MOVING
MOUNTAINS

About the Author

Michel Accad, MD, obtained his medical degree from the University of Texas Medical School in Houston, and completed his training in cardiology at the University of California, San Francisco. He practiced in diverse clinical settings before establishing his private practice in San Francisco.

Dr. Accad has previously made contributions to basic science research and therapeutic device development. Lately, his focus has been on the philosophical underpinnings of medical science and medical ethics. An avid reader and independent thinker, Dr. Accad has published provocative editorial and opinion pieces in the peer-reviewed literature. His commentaries on medical science, medical ethics, and healthcare economics appear on his blog AlertAndOriented.com.

MOVING MOUNTAINS

A Socratic Challenge to the Theory
and Practice of Population Medicine

Michel Accad, MD

2017
GREEN PUBLISHING HOUSE, LLC
College Station, Texas

Moving Mountains: A Socratic Challenge to the Theory and Practice of Population Medicine

ISBN 978-1-63432-030-6 (paperback)
ISBN 978-1-63432-031-3 (epub)
ISBN 978-1-63432-032-0 (pdf)
ISBN 978-1-63432-033-7 (mobi)

www.GreenPublishingHouse.com

To my wife Avelina for her unfailing support in all my quixotic projects. To our children Salim and Lucy, that they may experience a more humane healthcare system.

Acknowledgments

S ome of the material in this book first appeared several years ago as a series of blog posts. I am grateful to Dr. James Gaulte for encouraging me to turn that material into a book. I am especially thankful to Dr. Herbert L. Fred, my teacher, role model, and friend, for his kind and attentive review of the manuscript. I owe Herb an immense debt for indelibly impressing on me that medicine is not an abstraction, but a calling to care for and serve individual persons with specific needs and circumstances. I am also very thankful to Dr. Rocky Bilhartz for his support and suggestions, for his keen attention to detail, and for making the production of this book such an enjoyable collaboration.

Contents

"Hippocrates also pointed out that an inability to identify disease by species and genus leads to the failure of the doctor in his therapeutic aims.... That doctors need philosophy in order to employ their art in the right way seems to me to require no demonstration.... We must, then, practice philosophy if we are true followers of Hippocrates."

—Galen (129 - ca. 200/216 AD) in *The Best Doctor is Also a Philosopher*

Introduction

This book is an investigation into the theory of population medicine. In particular, it examines the theory of health and disease elaborated by Geoffrey Rose, the late British physician who is one of the intellectual founders of the population health movement. Rose's revolutionary ideas have been highly influential in public health circles. Today, the concepts epitomized in his theory have become guiding principles for healthcare systems around the world.[1]

---

[1] The online encyclopedia *Wikipedia* describes Rose as "an eminent epidemiologist whose ideas have been credited with transforming the approach to strategies for improving health." Although no one can properly take credit for the rise of the population health movement, which emerged in response to deep-seated factors (as will be discussed in the final chapter of this book), Rose is unique for the explicit attention he has given to the theoretical aspects of population medicine.

Inspired by Professor Peter Kreeft's didactic technique,[2] I have enlisted the help of Greek philosopher Socrates to cross-examine Rose's work. Using his characteristic method, Socrates subjects the ideas put forth in *The Strategy of Preventive Medicine* to a thorough but fair—and sometimes humorous—critique. The final chapter of the book offers my analysis of the broader context for Rose's theory, a context which looks to population medicine as a replacement for traditional individual care.

Throughout this book, direct quotes from Rose's work are presented in bold type. The exact sources for the quotes and for other citations in the text are provided in a bibliography section at the end the book.

WHO WAS GEOFFREY ROSE AND WHAT WERE HIS MAIN IDEAS?

Rose was born in 1926 and died prematurely in 1993 of pancreatic cancer shortly after publishing his only book, *The Strategy of Preventive Medicine*.[3] He studied medicine at Oxford in the 1950s and completed his training at St. Mary's Hospital in London under the tutelage of Sir George Pickering, one of the greatest clinical scientists of the time. Pickering's insights on the

---

[2] Professor Kreeft, from Boston College, has produced an entertaining series of introductory books on Western philosophy, e.g., *Socrates Meets Kant, Socrates Meets Descartes*, etc., published by Ignatius Press.

[3] All citations in the text refer to the 2nd edition of Rose's monograph, published in 2008 and titled *Rose's Strategy of Preventive Medicine*.

nature of hypertension were instrumental in shaping Rose's views about public health.

Rose became interested in cardiovascular epidemiology and preventive medicine early in his career. He made numerous methodological contributions to the development of diagnostic standards for coronary heart disease. He was principal investigator, along with the American epidemiologist Jeremiah Stamler, of the INTERSALT study, an important international investigation of the effect of dietary salt on cardiovascular health conducted across 52 different communities worldwide.

In 1985, Rose published his most acclaimed paper, "Sick Individuals and Sick Populations," in which he articulated his population strategy for public health. Initial expressions of his theory, however, had appeared in earlier articles, notably "Strategy for Prevention: Lessons from Cardiovascular Disease," published in 1981.

Three major tenets characterize Rose's theory of preventive medicine. The first tenet is that risk factors for disease in the population are distributed along continuous, bell-shaped curves. Because the risk imparted by risk factors is typically also continuous and graded, Rose believed that for any given disease, most clinical complications occur not in the minority of people at high-risk for the disease (the "tail" of the curve), but in the much larger number of subjects with risk factor profiles that are within the center of the distribution, closer to the mean.

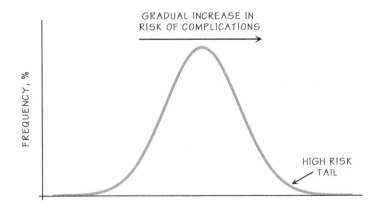

For example, the vast majority of cardiovascular complications is explained, not by the minority of patients with unequivocally high blood pressure or high cholesterol, but by the bulk of people with more moderate elevations in these risk factors. Accordingly, an effective public health intervention must aim to "shift" the entire bell-shaped curve down the risk scale, rather than "lop-off" the high-risk tail, since the latter approach would have no significant impact on public health statistics. Rose's approach has been widely adopted in disease prevention circles, as illustrated in the following graph adapted from the 7th Report of the Joint National

Committee on Prevention, Detection, Evaluation, and Treatment of High Blood Pressure:[4]

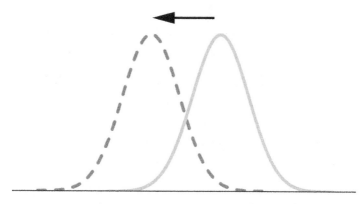

SYSTOLIC BLOOD PRESSURE (SBP)

PREDICTED REDUCTION IN MORTALITY FROM POPULATION-WIDE DROP IN SBP

REDUCTION IN SBP	STROKE MORTALITY	CORONARY MORTALITY	TOTAL MORTALITY
-2 (mmHg)	-6%	-4%	-3%
-3 (mmHg)	-8%	-5%	-4%
-5 (mmHg)	-14%	-9%	-7%

Beyond cardiovascular disease, Rose was convinced that his preventive strategy could apply to almost any condition: osteoporosis, obesity, hepatitis, neonatal death, depression, lead poisoning, and Down syndrome. According to his theory, all of these conditions display a risk-outcome relationship that lends itself perfectly to a population shifting strategy. Rose affirmed:

These concepts [of risk-outcome relationships] apply to the problems of prevention for almost

---

[4] (Chobanian et al. 2003).

every clinical specialty, as well as in occupational and environmental health and in the control of wider social problems.[5]

The second tenet of Rose's theory is that health and disease have a societal dimension, meaning that socio-economic conditions play a determining role in the prevalence of risk factors. Rose and Sir Michael Marmot, then a junior epidemiologist and now a highly influential authority on the question of "social determinants of health," were co-investigators of the famous Whitehall study. That study demonstrated that among British male civil servants, social grade and coronary mortality are inversely related, even after controlling for known coronary risk factors and access to medical care.

The results of the Whitehall study seem to support Rose's contention that health outcomes are influenced by emergent properties of societies and do not simply represent the cumulative effect of individual genetic factors, behaviors, and choices. For example, a man moving from Kyoto to Chicago will be subjected to the risk factor profile of his adoptive population, and his risk will vary accordingly, even without any conscious changes in his lifestyle or behavior.

The third tenet in Rose's theory derives naturally from the second: if social and economic determinants of disease are so important, medical activism must

---

[5] (Rose 2008, 110).

necessarily take on a political form. This is unequivocally stated in the last paragraph of Rose's book:

> **The primary determinants of disease are mainly economic and social, and therefore its remedies must also be economic and social. Medicine and politics cannot and should not be kept apart.**[6]

In that regard, Rose's philosophy is aligned with another dominant movement in public health, one whose primary goal is to eliminate health inequities, defined as "avoidable inequalities in health between groups of people within countries or between countries."[7] This movement found a home at the World Health Organization; at national public health agencies, such as the Center for Disease Control; within influential advisory organizations, such as the National Academy of Medicine; and in an increasing number of academic departments in the United States and abroad. These bodies have embraced Rose's theory unconditionally.

By prescribing a reduction in health inequities, Rose's theory echoes the thought of contemporary political philosophers, such as John Rawls's theory of social justice. But Rose's ideas provide social justice theories a needed scientific validation. And by broadening the scope of medical care so widely, his strategy allows

---

[6] (Rose 2008, 161).

[7] World Health Organization. Key concepts in the social determinant of health. Available at http://www.who.int/social_determinants/thecommission/finalreport/key_concepts/en/ accessed October 31, 2016.

medicine to become more openly a means of achieving political and economic change. At least, such is its hope.

Judging from his writing, which is simple, elegant, personal, and to the point, Rose was undoubtedly an erudite and a charming man. *The Strategy for Preventive Medicine* is short and easy to read. Its latest edition features a preface by two colleagues—one of whom is Michael Marmot—who describe Rose as a kind and honest person with a brilliant intellect and a contagious curiosity.

I have no doubt that Geoffrey Rose was an admirable man and that his interest for the betterment of mankind was genuine. But I also believe that his strategy, which aims at moving bell-shaped mountains of population characteristics according to the will of public health experts, amounts to a confused hodge-podge of propositions that are untenable on clinical, epidemiological, social, and ethical grounds—or on the basis of common sense alone.

1

Socrates Questions Rose About His Early Insights

THE SETTING:

A small, windowless conference room. Two bookcases containing out-of-date medical texts and journals line the walls. Small study tables are arranged "conference style" around the room. A large trash can filled with used coffee cups and with Styrofoam boxes emptied of take-out food gives off a rancid smell. The air is still and the ambient temperature stifling.

*Socrates, wearing a mantle, is seated at one end of the table arrangement. In front of him are his reading glasses, a copy of Rose's **The Strategy of Preventive Medicine**, and two other textbooks. Geoffrey Rose is seated at the corner to Socrates' right, wearing a beige shirt, navy striped tie, and a long white coat. In front of him is a short stack of diagrams and graphs.*

A handful of residents and students in crumpled short white coats occupy some of the remaining seats and manifest a vague interest in the conversation taking place. The room has a small exit door, guarded by an angel.

This is an internal medicine didactic conference held in purgatory.

SOCRATES: I've been asked to explore your theory of prevention, Geoffrey. As you know, I am more comfortable dealing with ethical and philosophical matters, but your work is not strictly concerned with facts of science. I have found it surprisingly stimulating. Are you ready for my cross-examination?

ROSE: I never imagined purgatory would be like this, Socrates. Are you going to demonstrate what St. Paul meant when he said that "fire will test the quality of each person's work?"

SOCRATES: That's the idea. Are you feeling the heat?

ROSE: Believe it or not, I don't mind being on the hot seat. I'm delighted to talk with you about my professional passion. I was forewarned, so I came prepared with all the charts and material that I need. Where shall we begin?

SOCRATES: Let's start at the beginning. How did you come to think so distinctly about the problem of "preventive medicine," as you call it?

ROSE: As I mentioned in my book, the starting point for me came from hearing Sir George Pickering explain his momentous insight on the nature of hypertension. It was in the mid-1950s and I was privileged to be his registrar at St Mary's Hospital.

SOCRATES: Pickering was an authority on hypertension, wasn't he?

ROSE: That's almost an understatement! He *was* the authority on hypertension, a man of towering intellect and a dominating personality. He had authored the textbook which, for two decades, was the main reference on high blood pressure. His famous debates with Lord Robert Platt—himself a prominent leader in medicine—were recorded in *The Lancet* where they captured the attention of the medical community for years.[8] Ultimately, the accumulated epidemiological and clinical research data vindicated Pickering's position.[9]

---

[8] Baron Robert Platt was a distinguished and influential physician with a particular interest in kidney diseases and hypertension. He became president of the Royal College of Physicians in 1957.

[9] *The Lancet* correspondence that constitutes the "Platt versus Pickering debates" was captured in a special text edited by Swayles (1985).

SOCRATES: What was Pickering's insight and how did it influence you?

ROSE: In those days, most of the medical community—Platt included—thought that hypertensive patients formed a distinct population. In other words, most doctors thought that the distribution of blood pressure in the population was "bimodal," as shown in this figure:

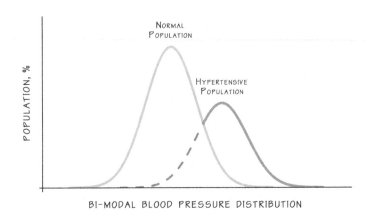

BI-MODAL BLOOD PRESSURE DISTRIBUTION

Pickering, on the other hand, believed that the distribution followed a bell-shaped curve with a single peak. He proposed that there is no threshold that distinguishes high blood pressure from normal blood pressure. In fact, in response to those who proposed a distinction between hypertension and "normotension," he was fond of saying that "the dividing line is nothing more or less than an artifact."[10] Given that the risk of cardiovascular events increases as the blood pressure increases, Pickering made the astonishing remark that this was the first instance of a disease that could be thought of as a *quantitative* rather than *qualitative* disorder.

Up until that time, the concept of disease was always understood in dichotomous, or binary terms: you either have tuberculosis or you don't; you either have diabetes or you don't, etc. Hypertension seemed entirely different, offering no clear cut demarcation between normal and abnormal. At the time, I was interested in the conditions that would lead some people to develop coronary disease, and it occurred to me that Pickering's observation could be applied to....

SOCRATES: Before we go any further, I would like to explore Pickering's assertion, if you don't mind. First of all, his idea seems commonplace to me. In my earthly days, we considered every disease as a quantitative imbalance of this or that humor: too much yellow bile makes people irritable, too much phlegm leads to apathy and depression. We inherited the general theory from the Egyptians, but Hippocrates and his followers solidified it. With that in mind, it seems that Pickering's insight was a step backward rather than a forward leap, don't you think?

ROSE: I never thought of it that way!

---

[10] (Pickering 1968, 178).

SOCRATES: Second, I don't fully see what must have seemed so novel about Pickering's idea, even in his time. After all, obesity was clearly preoccupying physicians in the 20th century. Is not corpulence a clear example of a quantitative disease?

ROSE: You're right and, in fact, Pickering was fond of saying that blood pressure is a quantity, just like height and weight. But no one really thought of obesity as a disease, really, unless it was obviously morbid. I mean, you wouldn't get people to worry about a few extra pounds, would you?

SOCRATES: You'd be surprised to know that a few short years after your death, the medical community would indeed begin to worry about any amount of extra weight. And I think your theory had a lot to do with that concern, but we'll get to that question in due time. Let's explore Pickering's idea a bit more.

ROSE: Let me then quote from the second edition of his textbook *High Blood Pressure*:

> The 'disease' essential hypertension, representing the consequences of raised pressure without evident cause, is thus a type of disease not hitherto recognized in medicine in which the defect is one of degree not of kind, quantitative not qualitative.
>
> The hypothesis just outlined has been greeted by medical scientists 'as a glimpse into the obvious,' and by physicians as 'dangerous nonsense because it is against accepted teaching.' It is apparently

difficult for doctors to understand because it is a departure from the ordinary process of binary thought to which they are brought up. Is it normal or abnormal, physiological or pathological, health or disease, good or bad? Quantity is not an idea that is as yet allowed to intrude. Medicine in its present state can count up to two but not beyond.[11]

SOCRATES: That's quite trenchant and seemingly irrefutable.

ROSE: I'd say! You should have seen the bafflement in the audience whenever Pickering shared his revolutionary insight at medical conferences. I, myself, felt that I was witnessing a true Copernican moment in medicine. And I quickly understood the ramifications of this discovery, for if you think about it....

SOCRATES: Before we get to the ramifications, let me probe these ideas a little bit more. I don't want to spend too much time on Pickering, but since his theory forms the backbone of your theory, I must point out that he himself seemed to waffle about "the nature of hypertension."

ROSE: Good Heavens! How could you say that? I was by his side when he began to articulate his argument and, for the next 20 years, he honed it into the sharpest intellectual sword, challenging anyone who would dare to duel with him. Apart from Platt, who was eventually defeated, few stood up to seriously question

---

[11] (Pickering 1968, 4).

Pickering because the emerging epidemiological data inexorably supported his idea: the blood pressure distribution in various populations never revealed any distinct dividing line, cohort studies showed that long-term outcomes were directly related to the baseline level of blood pressure, and clinical trials demonstrated that reduction in the blood pressure at any level of elevation improved long-term outcomes.

SOCRATES: I grant you all that, but if you read his textbook carefully, you will see him equivocating repeatedly.

ROSE: What?!

SOCRATES: Bear with me. For example, in the quote you just gave, he describes hypertension as being "a type of disease not hitherto recognized in medicine." Yet the opening paragraph of the very same chapter from which the quote is drawn makes an even sharper and snappier assertion that "[high blood pressure] is a sign not a disease,"[12] which contradicts the statement that hypertension is a "type of disease."

ROSE: Hypertension is both a sign and a disease. When the cause is known, as in Cushing's disease, it is a sign, but when the blood pressure is persistently elevated for no apparent reason, it is a disease that we call essential hypertension.

---

[12] (Pickering 1968, 1).

16

SOCRATES: I am aware of the distinction, but Pickering was still not very clear on that point. First of all, if there were two meanings for the term, he never clarified whether he was talking about the disease or the sign and, in fact, in the first edition of his textbook he even specified that the terms "high blood pressure," "hypertension," "hyperpiesia," and "hypertonia" were equivalent.[13]

Incidentally, William Evans was another prominent authority on hypertension, and he proposed to use one term—hypertonia—to refer to elevated pressure as a sign, and another term—hypertension—to indicate the disease.[14] But so far as I can tell, Pickering never made that distinction clear. In fact, here is another quote: "Essential hypertension represents little, and perhaps nothing more than the upper end of the distribution curve designated as essential hypertension at some arbitrary level such as 150 systolic, 100 diastolic."[15]

ROSE: Yes, absolutely, and it is based on this notion that I began to explore...

SOCRATES: Just a minute, my friend, I set the pace of the conversation here!

ROSE: Fair enough.

SOCRATES: When Pickering used the phrase "upper end of the distribution curve" he was talking about the

---

[13] (Pickering 1955, 6).
[14] (Evans 1957).
[15] (Pickering 1955, 6).

blood pressure distribution curve for the population at large, wasn't he?

ROSE: That's right.

SOCRATES: Which implies that there is no specific etiology for the disease operative in any individual patient, but rather, as Pickering would have it, a complex interaction of genetic and environmental factors that operate in the population at large.[16]

ROSE: Precisely.

SOCRATES: But, if that's the case, then it's like a disease that affects everybody, including those whose blood pressure is well below any "dividing line."

ROSE: Exactly! That's exactly the point! The entire curve is shifted!

SOCRATES: Except that Pickering was not comparing one curve versus another, and he did not really bring up the problem of an epidemic at all. He simply looked at the curve within a population, typically a Western country, and pointed to the upper end of the distribution as indicating essential hypertension. As far as he was concerned, essential hypertension was "unmasked" when Western populations started to live long enough to manifest its consequences. To him, the British population was essentially a normal population, although he also believed that environmental factors were at play in hypertension. So one obvious question

---

[16] (Pickering 1968, 290).

is: "In those days, would he have identified a Papuan man with a systolic blood pressure of 135 as hypertensive if that pressure level put him at the upper end of the distribution curve in Papua New Guinea?"

ROSE: You'd have to ask him that question yourself, Socrates!

SOCRATES: Maybe I will, because if he were consistent in his definition of hypertension, he would have had to classify such a person as having essential hypertension, which seems a little crazy to me. Furthermore, when it came to giving an explicit definition of what hypertension really is, Pickering shamelessly gave the "it depends" answer! He advised life insurance companies to ignore any definition based on cut-off points and, instead, told them to construct their actuarial tables on the basis of the baseline blood pressure value measured in a given patient.[17] In that regard, he made perfect sense: the risk of complications gradually increases as the blood pressure value rises.

For the physician dealing with a given patient, however, Pickering clearly side-stepped the answer, offering only some vague advice as to when treatment should be started and when a search for secondary causes would be warranted.[18] On the one hand, a certain cut-off blood pressure level—however arbitrary —must be selected if one is to "define" hypertension.

---

[17] (Pickering 1990, 14).
[18] Ibid.

On the other hand, Pickering exhorted everyone against using any specific number. In fact, he seemed particularly insistent on avoiding a focus on numbers so as not to frighten the patient needlessly. In the end, I think Pickering was ambivalent about how to deal with this "non-disease disease."

ROSE: I see your point Socrates, and I believe that my theory solves these problems very nicely.

SOCRATES: Very well, Geoffrey. I look forward to exploring your theory in detail, but we have covered enough ground for today. Let's leave that discussion for tomorrow's conference.

2

Rose Introduces Socrates to the Concept of a Sick Population

SOCRATES: The last time we spoke, we briefly covered Pickering's ideas on hypertension which, according to you, were instrumental in shaping your theory of prevention.

ROSE: Yes, Pickering's revolutionary proposal that there is no dividing line between hypertension and normotension; that the "disease" simply represents the tail end of the distribution curve; that physiology gradually creeps into pathology; and that "abnormal" is just too much of what looks otherwise normal. All of that really stimulated my thoughts. It occurred to me that his insight had implications far beyond the phenomenon of high blood pressure. In fact, **"disease is nearly always a quantitative rather than a categorical or qualitative phenomenon, and hence it has no natural definitions,"**[19] as I said in my book.

SOCRATES: Can you elaborate?

ROSE: If you don't mind I'll simply quote again from my book:

> **Infectious diseases in the population also come in all sizes, from obvious 'clinical' cases to symptomless infections that are only revealed by special laboratory tests. The clinical illness recognized as cancer is the infrequent end-stage of a series of common changes, beginning with minor cellular abnormalities (metaplasia) and ranging through more definitely premalignant change (dysplasia), localized (in situ) malignancy, and locally invasive disease. Interruption of cerebral blood flow can lead to a whole spectrum of consequences ranging from none at all, or symptoms too mild to come to medical attention, through a 'transient ischemic attack' (defined, quite arbitrarily, as a stroke that recovers with [sic] 24 hours), to a stroke with persistent disability or a dramatic and rapidly fatal illness.**[20]

---

[19] (Rose 2008, 43).
[20] Ibid.

And so forth, and so on. **"In most cases nature presents us with a process or continuum and not a dichotomy,"**[21] except in rare instances of congenital disorders determined by a single dominant gene with high penetrance, such as achondroplasia. There can be no argument about recognizing an achondroplastic dwarf: **"No one can have a 'touch of dwarfism.'"**[22]

SOCRATES: But according to you, a woman can have a touch of pregnancy, can she not?

ROSE: You're smiling and you may be trying to embarrass me! But tell me, Socrates, isn't it true, as I noted in my book, that even pregnancy develops in a series of steps?

SOCRATES (*putting on his reading glasses*): Well, Geoffrey, allow me to quote the entire passage:

> **Even pregnancy is not defined by nature, but rather it develops in a series of steps from the merely potential (a sperm swimming towards an ovum), through the stages of fertilized ovum, implantation in the uterus (apparently the legal definition), a biochemically detectable pregnancy, a clinically evident pregnancy, a recognizably human fetus, a viable fetus, and finally a live baby. The answer to 'When does a new life begin?' is thus an arbitrary issue, not a natural fact. Even the distinction between human and subhuman receives little support from nature.**[23]

---

[21] Ibid., 44.
[22] Ibid., 44.
[23] Ibid.

Holy Kalamata, Geoffrey! If you had uttered this in my days, I honestly couldn't say whether you'd have been dismissed as a fool or subjected to ostrakismós,[24] but I can also assure you that your academic career would have been categorically terminated!

ROSE: I have no doubt about that, Socrates. Thankfully, society has evolved in the last 2,500 years. We understand things much better now.

SOCRATES: I wouldn't be so sure, but let's leave aside your ideas about the beginning of life and about what differentiates a man from an ape, and let's just focus on your argument about diseases. It seems to me that you are offering a sort of medical version of Zeno's paradox.

ROSE: Come again?

SOCRATES: As you know, my contemporary Zeno of Elea argued that motion was illusion: to go from point A to point B you have to first reach the halfway point in-between, but before you reach the halfway point you have to reach the quarter-point mark, and before that, the eighth of the distance, and before that the sixteenth, and so forth to infinity. In the end you can never reach your destination. Since no one could find a flaw in his argument, he concluded that motion was an illusion. You seem to say that illnesses develop in a

---

[24] Ostracism. In ancient Athens, *ostrakon*, or pottery chards, were used as voting tokens in a procedure designed to expel from the community a citizen who was perceived as a threat.

continuous series of steps so that the notion of disease —as distinct from health—is an illusion.

ROSE: I never thought of it that way! That's not a bad analogy, Socrates.

SOCRATES: But do you know how Diogenes the Cynic refuted Zeno's argument?

ROSE: Yes, I know. Upon hearing it, he said nothing, stood up, and walked away. But Zeno's paradox is just an analogy for my argument, and all analogies have limitations. In this case, I am not making any argument about infinite steps, only small incremental steps that make it difficult to determine when health ends and disease begins.

SOCRATES: Fair enough, Geoffrey, but then it also seems to me that you are conflating the notion of disease severity with its presence or absence. Your contemporaries understood that a disease can sometimes be barely manifest, or may not even cause any symptoms at all. Sub-clinical cases do not invalidate the dichotomy between disease and health, do they?

ROSE: Socrates, my point seems to defy common sense, but I can assure you that it holds together very well if you view it from the right perspective.

SOCRATES: Enlighten me.

ROSE: The key is to look at things from a broader perspective. I am not really concerned with the illnesses and experiences of individual patients. I am conveying the viewpoint of an epidemiologist interested in the prevalence of disease in the population. A patient and his doctor are mainly attentive to diseases when these become manifest and action must be taken. For the epidemiologist, however, the whole spectrum of severity of illness must be taken into account, and not just the disease itself, but all the factors involved that predispose someone to disease.

Pickering's main insight about hypertension was that blood pressure is continuously distributed and that the risk of complications is related to the height of the pressure. He correctly stated that any dividing line is arbitrary as far as the definition of hypertension is concerned, but may be necessary for practical considerations, such as deciding when to begin therapy. I took his viewpoint a step further. I advanced that the disease is not determined by any arbitrary cut-off point selected along the distribution curve. I argued that a disease occurs when the whole distribution curve is shifted compared to where it should normally lie.

SOCRATES: So the disease is *in the population*?

ROSE: That's exactly right. That's the notion of "sick population," which I elaborated in my most cited paper.[25]

SOCRATES: So for you, the population *is* the patient?

---

[25] (Rose 1985).

ROSE: In a way, that's correct, at least from the standpoint of the epidemiologist.

SOCRATES: Thanks for the clarification, Geoffrey. This is indeed a revolutionary idea. We'll continue to explore it and examine what its implications might be at our next meeting. For now, I need some time to digest all of this.

3

Rose Explains the Fundamentals of His Theory

ROSE: Socrates, let me show you a graph that will help you better understand my theory. It comes from my best known paper, titled "Sick Individuals and Sick Populations."[26] On that graph, I have plotted the blood pressure distribution curve for two populations of middle-aged men: London civil servants and Kenyan nomads:

---

[26] (Rose 1985).

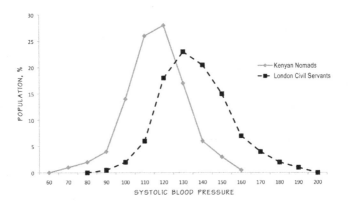

SOCRATES: I see that. Help me understand why that is helpful.

ROSE: You see, Socrates, if you consider each population separately and ask "why do some individuals have a higher blood pressure than others?", you may reasonably answer, as Pickering did, that variability in a large number of predominantly genetic factors accounts for this gradual, continuous curve. Pickering's position, as you recall, was that hypertension simply identifies the individuals at the higher tail-end of the distribution.

However, if you juxtapose the two population curves on the same chart, as I did here, and ask "**why is hypertension absent in the Kenyans and common in London?**"[27], you can see that the answer has everything to do with the position of the curve. As I

_____

[27] Ibid.

said in the paper, "**what distinguishes the two groups is nothing to do with the characteristics of individuals, it is rather a shift in the whole distribution—a mass influence acting on the population as a whole.**"[28] This is what happens to a given population when it migrates from a low prevalence setting to a high prevalence setting.

SOCRATES: All this is very interesting, Geoffrey. Let's take it one step at a time. When Kenyan cattle herders move to London, their blood pressure distribution moves to the right, is that correct?

ROSE: Yes, Socrates, the curve looks more like that of British civil servants.

SOCRATES: And the two curves—the old one and the new—will not have the exact same shape either, will they?

ROSE: Assuredly not. Blood pressure distribution curves in populations where hypertension is present are positively skewed, meaning that there's a larger number of individuals with a blood pressure to the right of the peak, as shown in this next figure, which is representative of the US population:[29]

---

[28] Ibid.
[29] Adapted from (Schwartz and Woloshin 1999).

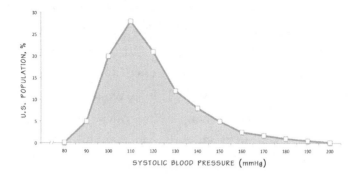

SOCRATES: And you think that the shift to a new distribution is primarily due to new environmental conditions?

ROSE: Exactly. It's only by looking at two different populations that the environmental effect can emerge. I have emphasized this point in the paper by saying that **"if everyone smoked 20 cigarettes a day, then clinical, case-control, and cohort studies alike would lead us to conclude that lung cancer was a genetic disease."**[30] You need a heterogeneity of exposures to be able to distinguish the effect of environmental or social causes.

SOCRATES: So tell me, Geoffrey, what is the cause of hypertension?

ROSE: Well, that's a pointed question! As you know, we have not discovered any one cause. Hypertension is a complicated condition in which multiple factors likely play a role. For example, the INTERSALT study, of which I was a principal investigator, demonstrated a

---

[30] (Rose 1985, 32).

positive relationship between salt excretion and the slope of age-related blood pressure increase, and this was seen by investigating 10,000 subjects in 52 centers worldwide. Within centers, the blood pressure itself was also positively related to salt excretion in a way that was partly independent of body mass index and alcohol intake, but the relationship was not present across centers.

SOCRATES: Geoffrey, I can hardly follow your jargon here. But from what I know, the role of dietary salt in hypertension is far from settled. Today, some authorities even suggest that salt restriction could be harmful![31] Would it be fair to say that the findings in your study were not as strong and clear-cut as many had hoped for, and that salt cannot be considered an obvious "cause" of hypertension?

ROSE: I'll grant you that. There is undoubtedly a multiplicity of factors that muddy the waters. For example, we did find a positive relationship between body mass index, alcohol intake, and high blood pressure.

SOCRATES: But the fact that no cause of hypertension has yet been firmly identified puts your theory in some doubt.

ROSE: What do you mean?

---

[31] Journalist Gary Taubes wrote an insightful review on the topic (Taubes, 1998). As of 2016, the controversy rages on, with some scientists claiming a very low salt diet may increase mortality rates.

SOCRATES: The graph that you produced comparing the Kenyan herders to the British civil servants is a striking one. As you showed, the entire blood pressure distribution curve can be shifted to the right. This suggests the presence of a single—or at most a few—strong factors that work on the entire population to cause the shift. Don't you find it odd that, so far, nothing of the sort has been identified?

ROSE: I disagree with you, Socrates. Granted, we have not identified simple factors to account for hypertension in the way we had hoped, but we have repeatedly demonstrated that when groups of individuals move from a society where the prevalence of hypertension is low to a society where the prevalence is high, the curve shifts. Similarly, when pre-industrial societies transition to become more urban and industrialized, the distribution curves for blood pressure and for other coronary risk factors also shift. That has to point to environmental factors associated with industrialization.

SOCRATES: The **"ills of affluence,"** [32] as you put it.

ROSE: Exactly.

SOCRATES: And when Kenyan cattle herders move to London, do they all experience an increase in blood pressure, or is it only a subset of them that the change affects?

---

[32] (Rose 2008, 36).

ROSE: That is hard to say. We have not conducted large scale studies measuring blood pressure in the same person at baseline and after migration to be able to answer your question factually. But if only a subset of immigrants were affected, we would likely see a second hump in the distribution curve after immigration. It would not be a smooth curve. My guess is that everyone experiences a rise in blood pressure but, in some, the rise may be greater than in others.

SOCRATES: Are you familiar with the work of Professor Chris McManus?

ROSE: As a matter of fact, we met on a couple of occasions.[33] He is a physician-scientist with a wide range of interests. He has conducted important cohort studies on medical students, but has also made important contributions to neuro-psychology. Why do you bring him up?

SOCRATES: As you yourself told me, part of the debate between Platt and Pickering concerned the blood pressure distribution in the general population and whether it had one peak or two. Pickering thought it had one peak and that essential hypertension was a multifactorial disease. Platt thought there were two peaks and that hypertension was a genetic disease with autosomal dominant transmission of variable penetrance.

---

[33] Chris McManus, personal communication.

ROSE: That's right.

SOCRATES: It is certainly true that Platt was incorrect regarding hypertension being an autosomal dominant genetic disease, but it is quite possible that he was correct regarding the blood pressure distribution having two peaks. As it turns out, when a distribution is positively skewed, the skew could be due to a distinct population with a small second peak that "hides" in the right side of the first peak. If that second peak is small, it may not show up distinctly, but the population that gives rise to it is responsible for the skew in the distribution. Here, I'll draw you a figure:

(Socrates puts on his reading glasses and sketches.)

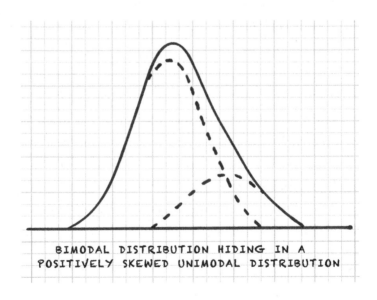

BIMODAL DISTRIBUTION HIDING IN A
POSITIVELY SKEWED UNIMODAL DISTRIBUTION

To be able to establish whether there is a hidden peak requires a large data set and sophisticated statistical analysis. In the early 1980s, professor McManus got hold of the only data set suitable for that purpose. It was a data set obtained in the mid-1950s by Norwegian epidemiologists. It was suitable because there was virtually no drug therapy for hypertension at that time. The data were not corrupted by the effect of treatment. It is one of the rare large epidemiological data set on blood pressure observed in the natural state, so-to-speak.

At any rate, McManus analyzed the data and came to the conclusion that Pickering may have been wrong after all, and that hypertension is, in fact, a distinct entity or rather, that people with hypertension form a distinct population.[34] As far as I know, his paper has not attracted much attention. It seems to me that the medical community is less interested in understanding hypertension and more interested in treating it, even if it does not necessarily understand what it is treating. But if McManus is correct, then there might be important personal factors that play a role in the development of the disease. Hypertension may not be solely due to widespread environmental or social conditions.

ROSE: That's very interesting Socrates, but McManus's findings were disputed by Schork and colleagues who

---

[34] (McManus 1983).

admittedly used a much smaller data set, but whose statistical analysis may have been more sophisticated than the one McManus used.[35] At any rate, the fact remains that when people move from underdeveloped nations to industrialized nations, their blood pressure increases. Whether all of them are affected or only a subset, I don't know and may never know, but the problem is serious enough that it warrants the approach that I propose and which I will now explain to you.

SOCRATES: Before we get there, I want to point out another weakness in your argument.

ROSE: What's the problem?

SOCRATES: You're missing an important piece of information.

ROSE: What would that be?

SOCRATES: What happens to British civil servants who become cattle herders in East Africa?

ROSE: What?! You're joking!

SOCRATES: I'm serious, or at least, the topic raised by the question is serious. According to your theory, the blood pressure curve should shift back to the left. Is there any evidence of that?

ROSE: As you can imagine, Socrates, there may be occasional eccentrics who give up modern comforts to adopt more primitive lifestyles, but there are not nearly

---

[35] (Schork, Weder, and Schork 1990).

enough of them to study their blood pressure before and after they leave Western civilization. So the answer is no, I do not have evidence one way or another to answer your question.

SOCRATES: But that's a very important point. It's not obvious to me that if there were enough hypertensive civil servants who traded their desk, their suburban home, and their predictable future for a vast expanse of wilderness and exposure to drought, injuries, or malaria, that we would see their blood pressure improve.

ROSE: I don't know that either, but to me, that point is contrived and unhelpful. The fact remains that millions of people are moving in the other direction, and their rate of hypertension, obesity, and diabetes is skyrocketing.

SOCRATES: Which leads me to my second objection.

ROSE: And what is *that*, Socrates?

SOCRATES: Don't be so surly, Geoffrey, and don't take this personally. I consider you a philosopher, not a sophist, willing to follow the truth, wherever it takes you. Our time is up anyway, so why don't we pursue this tomorrow morning?

4

Socrates and Rose Discuss Risk Factors and Diseases

SOCRATES: So Geoffrey, let's recap the main aspects of your theory that we have covered so far. If I may, I would summarize them as follows: First, from a population-based perspective, there is no dividing line between normal and pathological processes. A frequency distribution function for a disease can be envisioned as a smooth, continuous curve, provided that all the transition steps leading up to clinical manifestations are included, and not just the obviously symptomatic cases. As you said in your book, these are just **"the visible tip of the iceberg, which can neither be understood nor properly controlled if it is thought to constitute the entire problem."** [36] To follow your analogy, the bulk of the population is a "submerged mass" of people potentially at risk for complications.

ROSE: That's right, here's the graphic example:

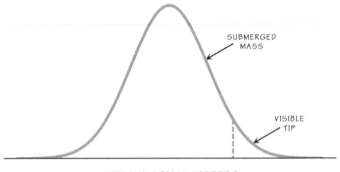

SUBMERGED MASS

VISIBLE TIP

EPIDEMILOGICAL ICEBERG

SOCRATES: Second, an epidemiologically important disease is a manifestation of a shift of the entire curve. For example, when people from a developing country migrate to the West, their blood pressure distribution curve shifts to the right and the number of cardiovascular complications rises dramatically.

ROSE: Yes.

---

[36] (Rose 2008, 45).

SOCRATES: Third, this shift in distribution must be explained by environmental and societal factors, since the genetic pool remains the same.

ROSE: I could not have said it better.

SOCRATES: Thank you. Can you walk me again through your explanation of why the distribution curve for any disease is a continuous curve? Show me your reasoning for something besides hypertension. How about making the case for hepatitis?

ROSE: All right, let me try again. Setting aside the rare genetic cases of hepatitis, such as Wilson's disease, do you agree that most forms of hepatitis are not genetically caused even if genetic factors undoubtedly play a role?

SOCRATES: Yes.

ROSE: For the sake of the discussion, let's lump all the different types of hepatitis together. I am not trying to establish diagnostic principles, but broad epidemiological ones. Now, do you also agree that many environmental and behavioral factors likely play a role in the development of liver disease, and that these factors can reinforce one another?

SOCRATES: I grant you that, too.

ROSE: Do you agree that hepatitis develops in stages; that the spectrum of severity is wide; and that fine gradations of hepatic disturbances could theoretically be identified along this spectrum, from near normal to a full-blown case of hepatic failure with jaundice and ascites?

SOCRATES: I do.

ROSE: Do you then agree that a patient who acquires hepatic disease moves from having a normal liver to having a malfunctioning one through a stage where the abnormality is imperceptible, unless the entire liver is available for examination under the most sensitive technique imaginable. The time course in the transition from normal to symptomatic disease may be quite rapid in the case of fulminant viral hepatitis, but it may be very slow in other forms of liver disease.

SOCRATES: I follow you.

ROSE: Imagine that you had in your possession a magic "hepatoscope" that could identify the slightest liver abnormality. If you could test every citizen on a given day, you'd be able to classify each one according to his position along the spectrum of subclinical and clinical abnormalities. The position would reflect the effect of all the relevant factors, genetic or environmental. That distribution curve would represent the totality of disease burden in the population.

SOCRATES: All right, but isn't it true that a large number of persons have a normal liver? Newborn babies and most children ought to be quite healthy in that regard.

ROSE: Yes, of course, but for any given age group, the same continuity in the distribution curve would hold, even though the shape of the curve might be different. Whatever age group you'd examine, the curve would be smooth and the bulk of "cases" would be asymptomatic. When a population is exposed to an unfavorable set of environmental factors, the entire curve will be shifted to the right, affecting dramatically the number of patients who develop clinical manifestations and are manifestly diseased.

SOCRATES: How is that?

ROSE: What do you mean, "How is that?" In the same way we showed it to be the case for blood pressure!

SOCRATES: But Geoffrey, there is a crucial distinction between the blood pressure example and what you've told me so far about hepatic disease. In the case of blood pressure, you (or Pickering) were plotting a frequency distribution curve for a *risk factor* which is known to be *predictive* of the risk of a future cardiovascular event. In the case of liver disease, you have produced a graph of the frequency distribution of the disease, subclinical or overt. But nothing here relates one's position along the abscissa to one's risk of becoming ill.

Let's take a hypothetical graph for the distribution of liver disease where we compare subjects A and B, both of whom are in the submerged, subclinical zone of the totality of hepatitis cases in the population. There is no compelling reason why subject B would necessarily have a greater risk of emerging into the tip of the iceberg (at position C) compared to subject A. Here, I'll draw you a figure:

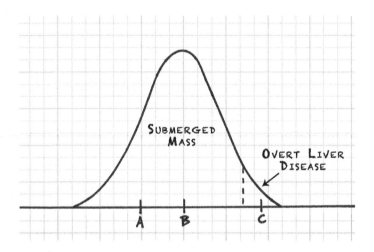

In the case of the blood pressure, the tail end of the curve is not a group of subjects that are necessarily ill but a group whose *risk* of becoming symptomatic is high. That has been well-established by long-term cohort studies. But in the curve that you've constructed for hepatitis, the tail end represents people with objective evidence of liver dysfunction. The two situations are distinct.

As I mentioned before, Pickering introduced some confusion when he was willing to call the tail end of the blood pressure curve the "disease" hypertension. He knew full well that finding a man with a blood pressure above 150/100 is no guarantee that he has objectively identifiable cardiovascular disease. Likewise, knowing that a man habitually goes to the pub at 10 o'clock in the morning is no guarantee that he actually has alcoholic liver disease. Conflating risk factor and disease is a basic conceptual error in my mind.

ROSE: I disagree. Everything else being equal, I'd rather have a blood pressure of 110/70 than a blood pressure of 150/100, and most people would, too. So high blood pressure is itself a kind of disease, just like consistently drinking too much alcohol is a kind of disease. My general point is that the burden of disease is born by the overwhelming majority of people with risk factors or with subclinical disease. As I said in my book:

Preventive medicine should be concerned with the whole spectrum of disease and ill health, both because all levels are important to the people concerned and because the mild can be the father of the severe.[37]

SOCRATES: I'm not sure to what extent people are concerned with things they are unaware of. More importantly, it seems you're putting the cart in front of the horse, Geoffrey. This prognostic relationship

---

[37] Ibid.

between subclinical disease and clinical disease, or the truth about **"the mild being the father of the severe,"** as you say, is what you need to demonstrate. You cannot assume that the relationship exists.

It is quite possible that for many diseases, the relationship is not graded and continuous but subject to threshold effects or even reverse relationships. In fact, such may even be the case for blood pressure. Shortly after you died, some scientists observed that elderly people who have a very low blood pressure may be at higher risk of future cardiac complications.[38] Besides, in the case of subject B mentioned earlier, the exposure to risk factors may have been heavier than in the case of subject A at the time they were both examined, but B's exposure may change over time. He or she may heal, and as time goes by, B may have a burden of subclinical disease that is less than that of A's.

ROSE: Socrates, I focused on the topic of exposure and risk, and I fully elaborated on the possible relationships. I understand the problem well, and this is what I said:

---

[38] Socrates refers to the so-called "J-curve" phenomenon, which owes its name to the shape of the variable-outcome curve when plotted on a graph. In elderly people, there is a sharp rise in coronary mortality rates as the blood pressure increases, but there is also another rise—albeit less pronounced—when the blood pressure is at the low end of the spectrum.

Two issues concerning the shape of the dose-effect relationship are critical for preventive policy. How much of the burden of ill health is compressed within an identifiable group where high exposure carries a high personal risk? Is there an exposure threshold below which risk is negligible and can be ignored?

Both these questions require us to look at the whole ranges of both exposure to causes and health outcomes. Where research has proceeded in this way, it has often appeared that there is a graded threshold-free relation between cause and effect....[39]

SOCRATES: But earlier in the same chapter, you highlighted how difficult it is to empirically identify the exposure-risk relationship. You even mentioned a study that you personally led in which you examined the effects of radiation on 39,000 subjects who were followed for 16 years. You admitted that, at the study's end, you couldn't say "**whether the International Commission on Radiological Protection had set a standard which on the one hand was too high, or on the other hand might have been 15-fold too low.**"[40] You described as "mind boggling" the scale and complexity of studies that aim to measure dose-effect relationships or identify threshold effects.

---

[39] (Rose 2008, 62).
[40] Ibid., 55.

ROSE: Yes, there are some difficulties. In many cases, however, we are able to identify a graded relationship between exposure and risk. Take the relationship between dietary fat, serum cholesterol, and heart disease.

SOCRATES: Geoffrey, you really need to be brought up to date![41]

ROSE: I heard that the story is more complicated than what we initially believed, but I think you are getting bogged down in technicalities and not seeing the big picture, Socrates.

SOCRATES: Let's go back to the big picture, then. Your idea is that from a public health standpoint, it is more beneficial to reduce exposure to risk factors in the entire population than to focus on the small group of patients at high-risk of developing clinical disease.

ROSE: I carefully examine both approaches, weigh the pros and cons of each, and draw my own conclusions at the end of the book.

SOCRATES: Let's then examine what you have to say about the "high-risk" approach tomorrow.

ROSE: I need that break, you're exhausting me!

---

[41] Witness the cover article for the June 12, 2014, issue of *TIME* magazine titled "Eat butter. Scientists labeled fat the enemy. Why they were wrong."

5

Rose Explains the "High-Risk" Strategy for Prevention

SOCRATES: Hello, Geoffrey, did you get some rest?

ROSE: I did, thank you, but I would certainly like to pick up the pace and not get bogged down into ridiculous minutiae.

SOCRATES: Fine. You are now going to share with me your perspective on what you call the "high-risk" strategy of prevention. If I understand it correctly, this strategy essentially aims at "lopping off the tail" of the distribution curve.

ROSE: That's essentially it. It amounts to identifying and treating people who are at high-risk of developing disease, and those who have no symptoms but objectively detectable abnormalities, i.e., those with subclinical disease.

For example, the approach would aim to identify all people whose blood pressure is above a certain arbitrary value, and treat them to bring the pressure down into the so-called "normal range," as described in this next figure:

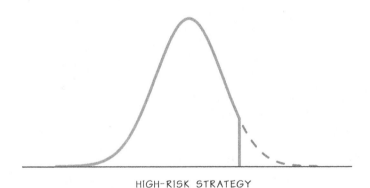

HIGH-RISK STRATEGY

SOCRATES: You didn't come up with that strategy, did you?

ROSE: Oh no! The high-risk approach has been around for a long time. This is the strategy that doctors and patients are most accustomed to.

Decades ago, for example, we used to screen for infectious diseases like tuberculosis in this way. Today, we screen for malignant or pre-malignant tumors with mammography or colonoscopy.

The strategy of identifying high-risk individuals by way of screening was described in detail in a landmark paper by Jungner and Wilson, published by the World Health Organization in 1968.[42] That paper was beautifully written and remains highly relevant today, especially in light of what we have discussed so far.

SOCRATES: Tell me more.

ROSE: The authors discussed screening in the context of the two possible situations you and I have talked about. They constructed two schematic distribution curves for disease variables: one for those that have a bimodal distribution, and one for those that have a unimodal distribution:

---

[42] (Jungner and Wilson, 1968).

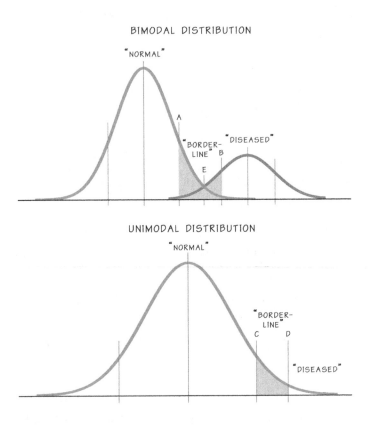

SOCRATES: According to what you told me last time, you think that most disease variables can be conceptualized as following a unimodal distribution.

ROSE: That's correct, we don't need to worry about bimodal distributions. Jungner and Wilson noted that in the case of unimodal distributions, the number of "borderline" cases (those whose screening test result falls between C and D in the bottom figure above) can be larger than the number of cases of actual disease (to the right of D). Besides, in a unimodal distribution, both C and D are essentially arbitrary. For example, one might say that 135/80 represents "borderline" hypertension, and that 150/100 represents "actual" hypertension. But in truth, neither number has any physiological or pathological reality. So, depending on how one selects these cut-off points for screening, a very large number of subjects could fall in the "borderline" category. These individuals will either be misclassified as having the disease or will need to undergo additional testing.

SOCRATES: And for you, that's a problem.

ROSE: Naturally. Mild or borderline cases, when considered individually, tend to have a good prognosis. As I said in my book:

> **[In the Medical Research Council trial of treatment for mild hypertension,] the relative risk of stroke increased steeply with increasing blood pressures, and treatment effectively reduced it, but for any one individual the absolute risk was low, and overall it needed 850-person-years of treatment in order to prevent one stroke.[43]**

On the other hand, if you move your cut-off numbers to minimize the borderline cases, you may avoid over-treating bystanders but you will miss treating patients headed toward complications.

---

[43] (Rose 2008, 83).

SOCRATES: That's frustrating.

ROSE: That's right. And another issue with identifying a large number of borderline cases is that they will frequently fall prey to "medicalization."

SOCRATES: What do you mean?

ROSE: Consider this passage from my book:

> **The man who went to see his doctor because he had a pain in his neck walked away from that encounter bearing a label of 'hypertensive patient,' which he must now wear for the rest of his life. Having hitherto perceived himself as healthy, he now has to see himself as someone needing to take pills and to see the doctor regularly. He was, he thought, normal; now he is a patient. This may be unavoidable and justified by the benefits, but it is a major cost.[44]**

SOCRATES: I think you refer here to what the medical literature calls the "labeling effect."

ROSE: Exactly. And there is good evidence that labeling carries with it a number of negative consequences: people start acting sick, they start experiencing symptoms when they had none before the label was applied, they miss days at work, etc.

SOCRATES: So, if I can summarize your point of view at this juncture, you think that most diseases follow a unimodal distribution. Therefore, a preventive strategy that aims to identify high-risk individuals by way of

---

[44] Ibid., 81.

some kind of screening protocol is problematic because setting the cut-off points for borderline cases and for "true" cases is arbitrary and can lead to either over-diagnosing the healthy or under-diagnosing the sick.

ROSE: That's a nice summary.

SOCRATES: And your strategy avoids this problem?

ROSE: I believe it does.

SOCRATES: Before we go there, let's finish our exploration of the high-risk strategy. Jungner and Wilson gave recommendations for a good screening strategy, didn't they?

ROSE: That's right. These are tabulated as follows:

(1) The condition sought should be an important health problem.
(2) There should be an accepted treatment for patients with recognized disease.
(3) Facilities for diagnosis and treatment should be available.
(4) There should be a recognizable latent or early symptomatic stage.
(5) There should be a suitable test or examination.
(6) The test should be acceptable to the population.
(7) The natural history of the condition, including development from latent to declared disease, should be adequately understood.
(8) There should be an agreed policy on whom to treat as patients.
(9) The cost of case-finding (including diagnosis and treatment of patients diagnosed) should be

economically balanced in relation to possible expenditure on medical care as a whole.

(10) Case-finding should be a continuing process and not a "once and for all" project.

SOCRATES: Do you agree with these recommendations?

ROSE: Yes, I do. In my book, I specifically elaborated on recommendations (2), (3), and (9). As far as recommendation (2) is concerned, I stressed that we should go after *reversible* risk factors, not risk factors about which we cannot do anything. Furthermore, I emphasized that **"policy decisions must therefore be founded on absolute, not relative, risk estimates, and they should take account of those other factors which modify the risk of a particular exposure."**[45] For example, treating an elevated cholesterol level in a patient with normal blood pressure and no other risk factors offers a trivial benefit to the individual or the population.

SOCRATES: I think this point is now more commonly accepted in academic circles, although that was not the case when you wrote your book. You were ahead of your time in that regard. What about recommendation (3), that "facilities for diagnosis and treatment should be available?"

ROSE: It seems obvious to me that if one is going to adopt a screening strategy to identify high-risk patients, it is imperative that resources be put in place

[45] Ibid., 74.

to offer the appropriate therapy. Experience shows repeatedly that effective interventions require education, involvement of the practitioner, and sustained follow-up. I stated:

> **A policy of mass screening for risk identification presupposes a medical care system which is able to provide continuity of long-term personal care for everyone. This is a major obstacle to effective preventive care in countries such as the USA, which lack a general practitioner system covering the whole population. In Britain, and in other countries fortunate enough to possess such a system, at least the potential is there for long-term preventive care, but its realization requires substantial additional investment in staff, training, and organization.**[46]

SOCRATES: You'll be interested to learn that authorities in the United States are now actively trying to emulate the British system by establishing so-called "patient-centered medical homes," where the primary care physician is in charge of orchestrating preventive services.[47]

ROSE: Hallelujah!

---

[46] Ibid., 71.

[47] "Patient-centered medical homes" is a term that refers to a practice arrangement whereby care is orchestrated by a primary care physician working in association with a hospital-linked "Accountable Care Organization," with the expectation that the arrangement will improve quality and reduce costs. Such practice arrangements are encouraged by the reforms associated with the Affordable Care Act of 2010.

SOCRATES: But don't be too optimistic. Neither the British National Health Service nor the American system seem to be in a financial position to provide the resources that you think are necessary to carry out preventive services as you envision.

ROSE: As I see it, that's unfortunate and short-sighted.

SOCRATES: What about recommendation (9)? How should costs be considered?

ROSE: I remark that *selective* screening is always more cost-effective than *mass* screening. I state:

> **Simple and readily available information may often indicate that risk is more likely to be found in one group than another. This can make it profitable to plan a two-staged process in which one looks for high-risk individuals only within a high-risk sector of the population.**[48]

SOCRATES: That makes perfect sense to me. All-in-all, Geoffrey, I don't find you to be all that set against a high-risk strategy for prevention.

ROSE: Not at all. I even said that **"preventive medicine must embrace both, but, of the two, power resides with the population strategy."**[49] The high-risk strategy has some important benefits but also some shortcomings.

---

[48] (Rose 2008, 71).
[49] Ibid., 49.

SOCRATES: We have exposed some of the shortcomings. What are the benefits?

ROSE: I identify the main benefit of a high-risk strategy in the fact that "**the intervention is appropriate to the individual.**"[50] The high-risk approach "**avoids interference with those who are not at special risk.**"[51]

SOCRATES: That is except for the borderline cases which, depending on how you set up your cut-off points, could be a very large number of people.

ROSE: That's true, but public health experts are likely to make reasonable decisions regarding the selection of cut-off points.

SOCRATES: I would not be so optimistic. In the case of hypertension, for example, the debate regarding where those cut-off points should be set seems to get more heated by the hour. European experts want them set one way, Americans another, yet they are all looking at the same data. What's more, a new study gets published every so often that sends everyone into a tailspin.[52]

There is another aspect of this high-risk strategy that bothers me. As you yourself recognized, clinicians have difficulty predicting the clinical course that any given person will follow, particularly when it comes to

---

[50] Ibid., 77.

[51] Ibid., 78.

[52] For an overview of the difficulties and controversies that arise from defining high blood pressure according to cut-off points, see (Accad and Fred, 2010).

chronic conditions like coronary disease or hypertension. In recommendation (7), Jungner and Wilson stated that "the natural history of the condition, including development from latent to declared disease, should be adequately understood." It seems to me that by this criterion, much of cardiovascular disease would be disqualified from becoming the target of a screening strategy.

ROSE: That's crazy! We have had great success with our screening procedures for hypertension, serum cholesterol, smoking, and so forth. Coronary disease mortality has plummeted in the last 30 years, and stroke is clearly on the decline.

SOCRATES: I don't dispute that, but how do you know that the decline is due to a widespread screening strategy?

ROSE: Do you mean to say that the decline has been spontaneous? That's preposterous!

SOCRATES: I'm just trying to be cautious. As you well know, correlation is not causation. Besides, the temporal association between the decline in mortality and screening may not be as clear as you think. You may not be familiar with the work of Professor William Rothstein, a medical historian at the University of Maryland. He published a book on the history of risk factors in 2003, about a decade after you died.[53] He made a very interesting observation.

ROSE: Tell me about it.

SOCRATES: By carefully analyzing vital statistics from life insurance policyholders, he saw that the onset of the decline in coronary heart disease mortality occurred earlier than is commonly thought. The standard account is that the decline began in the mid 1960s. By then, Ancel Keys had made it on the cover of *TIME* magazine,[54] the first report of the Framingham study had been published,[55] and the Surgeon General's warning against the dangers of cigarette smoking had been issued.[56] What Rothstein actually discovered is that in the healthier segments of the populations, the onset of the decline in coronary mortality occurred earlier, probably in the late 1950s, and *preceded* any measurable decline in the prevalence of risk factors within these same groups. I'll give you an exact quote

---

[53] (Rothstein 2003). This text by Professor Rothstein is a must read for anyone interested in cardiovascular epidemiology and public health.

[54] January 13, 1961. Keys was a celebrated epidemiologist and the most influential proponent of the diet-lipid hypothesis as the major cause of the coronary disease epidemic.

[55] July 1, 1961, issue of the *Annals of Internal Medicine*. With that publication, the Framingham study introduced the concept of "risk factor" into the medical lexicon. It identified age, male sex, elevated serum cholesterol level, and high blood pressure as the major risk factors for coronary artery disease (Kannel et al. 1961).

[56] The 1964 report by the Surgeon General was ranked among the top news stories of that year. See the Center for Disease Control's "History of the Surgeon General's Report on Smoking and Health," available at http://www.cdc.gov/tobacco/data_statistics/sgr/history/.

from his book: "These data demonstrate conclusively that changes in personal risk factors were not responsible for the secular decline in coronary heart disease mortality and morbidity rates."[57]

ROSE: Hmmm.

SOCRATES: There is also a chart produced by the US Center for Disease Control which caught my attention. In 1999, they issued a brief report titled "Achievements in Public Health: Decline in Death from Heart Disease and Stroke—United States, 1900-1999."[58] Here is the graph:

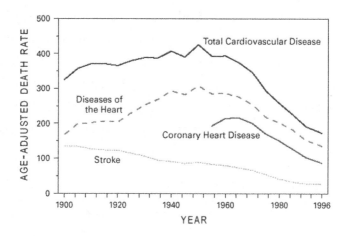

As you can see, stroke mortality has been steadily declining since the beginning of the twentieth century,

---

[57] (Rothstein 2003, 353).
[58] Center for Disease Control. Morbidity and Mortality Weekly Review. 1999, 48:649-56. Available online at http://www.cdc.gov/mmwr/preview/mmwrhtml/mm4830a1.htm.

with no change in the slope of the trend before and after the identification of cardiovascular risk factors.

ROSE: Socrates, you don't mean to say that we should now tell people they can neglect their blood pressure and eat, smoke, and drink to the heart's content? That's crazy!

SOCRATES: I'm not saying that, Geoffrey. There is also clearly a correlation between good health habits and increased life expectancy. But public health interventions bring with them a cost which Jungner and Wilson were aware of in 1968, and which nowadays seems completely overlooked. They specifically say: "In enthusiastically attacking disease at an early stage, the Hippocratic principle ...*primum no nocere*, should not be neglected."

ROSE: Socrates, Hippocrates was your contemporary and I suspect that you know full well he did not enunciate the principle in that way.[59]

SOCRATES: Touché! But my point remains that when a screening policy is established, some committee of experts somewhere decides what risks and benefits justify the given approach. I suspect that your man

---

[59] According to the online encyclopedia *Wikipedia,* the well-known phrase may have emerged in the nineteenth century. The closest rendition found in the Hippocratic corpus is "The physician must... have two special objects in view with regard to disease, namely, to do good or to do no harm," which is a more realistic principle since the risk of harm is inherent in any medical intervention. See https:// en.wikipedia.org/wiki/Primum_non_nocere accessed October 12, 2016.

walking into the doctor's office with a stiff neck is not involved in that decision.

ROSE: Well, what do you propose, Socrates?

SOCRATES: You could at least ask your man if he wishes to have his blood pressure taken, his cholesterol measured, or his seat belt behavior scrutinized. You could spend the time educating him about his *a priori* risk, and explain to him how that risk would be modified by the screening test, what harm might ensue from a borderline finding, and what the imprecision in predicting outcome really is. In other words, you could put into place resources to educate patients *before* actually applying the test. That would really be an approach adapted to the individual, since it would take into account his or her personal risk tolerance.

ROSE: But that's completely impractical! And besides, most patients would defer the decision to the doctor. You know the chime: "You know best, doctor!"

SOCRATES: If they say that, then you may have the ethical leeway to make the decision on behalf of the patient. But patients may not defer decision-making to the doctor as often as you would think. It is true that decades ago, a doctor's opinion was viewed as sacrosanct. Today, however, many people expect to be involved in medical decisions. They may also seek the counsel of others. Have you heard of something called the internet? It is a remarkable vehicle for disseminating information and for sharing experiences and opinions.

ROSE: I don't know what the internet is, but if the scenario you outline materializes, it is likely that very few people would accept screening, since individual risk is always very low. This would completely reverse all the gains we have made over the last 30 years!

SOCRATES: Who knows, Geoffrey? Many people may actually decide that it is worthwhile to get screened. Some sociologists have remarked that risk avoidance is a mark of affluent societies, so screening could appeal to people even if they understand themselves to be at low risk.

ROSE: Let's not get carried away with wishful thinking, Socrates. Let's rather agree that a preventive strategy based on screening for high-risk individuals is less than optimal. Why don't we explore my "population" strategy instead?

SOCRATES: Excellent idea, Geoffrey, but let's leave this for tomorrow.

6

Rose Gives Specific Examples of the Population Approach

SOCRATES: Well, Geoffrey, let's get into the meat of your population approach.

ROSE: It's about time!

SOCRATES: As we previously discussed, the main idea is to try to shift the distribution curve in a direction that matches the variable-to-risk relationship.

ROSE: That's right. If the risk of complications increases as the value for the variable gets higher—as is the case for the blood pressure—then we would want to shift the entire curve in a decreasing, right-to-left fashion, as shown in this next figure:

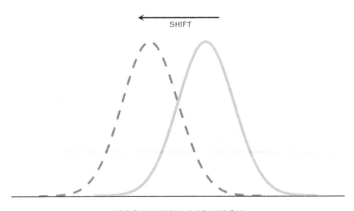

POPULATION STRATEGY

SOCRATES: In chapter 6 of your book, you first make the point that a change in the population mean of a given characteristic will be accompanied by a change in the prevalence of clinical cases or, as you put it, of "deviants."

ROSE: That's right. We have touched on this before, but what this signifies is that a favorable shift in the distribution curve will affect the tail so that the number of symptomatic or overt cases will be reduced. We were able to show this in the INTERSALT study. To give you an example, we showed that as the mean body weight in the population declines, the prevalence of obesity also declines.[60] We found a similar linear relationship between mean blood pressure and prevalence of hypertension, and between mean salt excretion and prevalence of high sodium intake. We also showed that the relationship holds for mean alcohol intake and the prevalence of heavy drinking. Here is the graph depicting the relationship between mean body weight and prevalence of obesity in the population:

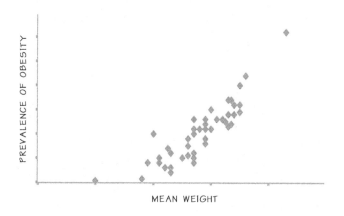

SOCRATES: Is this plot truly an illustration of your population approach? To me, the graph indicates the mean weight and the prevalence of obesity for many

---

[60] (Rose and Day 1990).

different populations. It shows that in countries where the mean weight is low, the prevalence of obesity is low. Conversely, where the mean weight is high, the prevalence of obesity is high. But the graph does not show that if you intervene to lower the mean weight *of a given population*, i.e., if you shift the curve, the prevalence of obesity will, in fact, decline. That's your hope, correct?

ROSE: That's correct, but I find it difficult to imagine that the prevalence of disease would not decline from shifting the curve.

SOCRATES: That may be true, but it is important to maintain clarity between what is hypothetical and what is established. More importantly, Geoffrey, it seems to me that the graph is rather trivial.

ROSE: What do you mean, trivial?

SOCRATES: Whether you look at blood pressure, salt excretion, or body weight, you are talking about variables that are known to follow a more-or-less normal distribution.[61] It stands to reason that any shifting of the whole curve *en bloc* will also lower the frequency of values at the high end of the curve. You're doing nothing more than highlighting a well-known

---

[61] To be precise, most biological distributions follow a "log-normal" distribution, but the point made by Socrates stands.

property of normally-distributed data. In fact, some scholars have criticized you for this.[62]

ROSE: Well, I thought it was important nevertheless to stress this relationship, as there are many who view the population approach to prevention with a great deal of skepticism. I provide other examples in that chapter, notably some about mental health. I show that if we examine the prevalence of mental disease as measured by a reliable psychiatric screening questionnaire, we also see that the distribution is "**continuous, with a single mode and no suggestion of any break between 'cases' and 'normals,' implying that the commoner forms of mental illness are a quantitative and not a categorical disorder.**"[63] The same goes for senile dementia.

SOCRATES: I've been thinking about these mental illness examples, Geoffrey, and I can think of a reason why the results would necessarily favor your hypothesis.

---

[62] A searing critique to the paper above, written by Petr Skrabanek—the iconoclastic physician, scientist and author of *Follies and Fallacies in Medicine*—was published as a letter to the editor in *BMJ*. The opening sentence reads as follows: "The premises on which Professor Geoffrey Rose and Mr. Simon Day build their argument that the normal majority must change is fallacious, their reasoning faulty, and their evidence irrelevant. The only common denominator to their data seems to be the trivial observation that shifting population means also shifts the tails of the distribution" (Skrabanek 1990). Another critical letter was written by Swiss statistician Stephen J Senn, then employed at Ciba-Geigy, and now professor at the University of Glasgow (Senn 1990). Rose did not answer these two negative letters but replied to two other letters that were more positive.
[63] (Rose 2008, 105).

ROSE: And what reason is that, Socrates?

SOCRATES: Psychiatric disorders are typically described in terms of symptoms, feelings, and behaviors that are common but for some reason or another, the manifestation is at the extreme end of the spectrum: too much sadness, too much anxiety, too much alcohol intake, too much egotism, etc. These are by *definition* quantitative disorders and, therefore, they are naturally well-suited to fit your model.

ROSE: And what's wrong with that?

SOCRATES: If you only pick examples which, by definition, are quantitative disorders, you are making an easy claim for your theory. Case in point: the examples of mental illness you chose are all defined according to a scoring system. What other examples do you provide?

ROSE: I elaborate further on a population-wide strategy to decrease cardiovascular disease rates by lowering blood pressure and cholesterol values for all members of the population, but we have discussed this at length already. I also show how the population approach could be applied to the problem of infants with low birth weight, but I give this example primarily to acknowledge that there are caveats of which we should be mindful. The relationship between birth weight and infant survival is U-shaped, meaning that there is a possibility of harm at both ends of the spectrum. So, we should be cautious about introducing interventions that will shift the birth weight distribution curve one way or another. Furthermore, I note that most of the mortality increases seem to be borne by a separate population of babies with a very small birth weight. I conclude: **"To reduce the size of this small but critical group calls for a small and more focused approach."**[64]

SOCRATES: Aren't you essentially saying that birth weight follows a bi-modal distribution? And are you not advocating here a "high-risk" approach for prevention?

ROSE: Hmmm. You may be right about that. But, I also add that **"differences in birth weight are ultimately linked to social inequalities."**[65]

SOCRATES: What does it have to do with your population strategy for prevention?

ROSE: We haven't yet touched upon the social determinants of health, which I will discuss later in the book. But social scales are graded and they influence health. If one is serious about public health, one has to seriously think about all dimensions of risk factors.

SOCRATES: Let's not get side-tracked, Geoffrey. We'll address the social determinants in due time. What's the next example of your population strategy?

ROSE: The next example describes how health and nutrition at an early age are related to the risk of

---

[64] Ibid., 115.
[65] Ibid., 115.

cardiovascular disease later in life. This is another example of how social inequalities could impact health.

SOCRATES: If you are trying to make the case that poverty is a risk factor for ill health, you may be breaking down open doors! What's your next example?

ROSE: Down syndrome. You won't accuse me of picking a quantitative disorder, here, will you?

SOCRATES: Certainly not, but I'm curious to see how your strategy will unfold.

ROSE: Very simply. As it turns out, a study in England and Wales showed that "**if special screening tests are confined to mothers aged 35 and over, then one cannot hope to identify much more than a quarter of the affected pregnancies [given that women age 20-29 represent the most fertile segment].**"[66]

SOCRATES: Do you suggest screening *all* mothers?

ROSE: That would be one option, but that's not what I am suggesting. Another option is to lower the average maternal age.

SOCRATES: Force mothers to have babies sooner?

ROSE: Of course, not. The role of the public health investigator is to inform the public about the relationships between risk factor and illness, but freedom of choice must be maintained. Some societies may choose to institute policies that encourage women

---

[66] Ibid., 117.

to have children at a younger age without being overly coercive.

SOCRATES: That's very good, Geoffrey. Stay above the fray and eschew responsibility! Is that all you have?

ROSE: There's more. I also discuss the results of a study that showed a steep inverse linear relationship between bone mass and incidence of fractures. The study allows us to estimate that a 12 percent increase in average bone density in the population could result in a 20% decline in fractures. This can be achieved by controlling recognized risk factors for low bone mass. I add that **"the use of hormone replacement in women at and after menopause could add further to the protection, but only for as long as it continues to be taken."**[67]

SOCRATES: Hmmm. You might be interested to know that your suggestion was widely adopted, but the outcomes were not as you might have hoped.

ROSE: Hormones did not prevent osteoporotic fractures?

SOCRATES: Not only that, but hormone replacement increased rates of cardiovascular catastrophes and of certain forms of cancer.[68]

ROSE: Oh my!

SOCRATES: Yes, "Oh my!" Do you have any other examples?

ROSE: My last example concerns radiation exposure.

---

[67] Ibid., 123.
[68] (Roussow et al. 2002).

SOCRATES: I read that part, so let me quote you directly. In regards to the dose-response relationship between radiation and cancer you state: "**Although no one can be certain, it is widely assumed that the dose relationship between radiation exposure and cancer is threshold free and linear.**"[69] Unfortunately, Geoffrey, what was "widely assumed" in your days would be widely in doubt a few years later. Some scientists now even claim that low doses of radiation are necessary for good health.[70]

ROSE: Interesting! But that doesn't change the basic principles of my theory. Once we know more about the exposure-risk relationship, we can adjust the public health recommendations accordingly.

SOCRATES: By then, it might be too late!

ROSE: We have serious public health problems on our hands, Socrates, so let's not have paralysis by analysis! Worrying about improbably small chances of causing harm is not the way to move forward, especially when many of our health woes can be ameliorated by simply improving social conditions.

---

[69] Ibid., 124.

[70] The "linear no-threshold" doctrine, according to which any amount of radiation is harmful, is now believed to be false or very doubtful by a growing number of scientists. See, for example, (Tubiana et al. 2009). For a discussion of the position that a small amount of radiation is necessary for health, see David Warmflash's article published April 6, 2015, on the blog of the *Discovery Magazine*, "Could Small Amounts of Radiation Be Good for You? It's Complicated," available at http://blogs.discovermagazine.com/crux/2015/04/06/small-radiation/.

SOCRATES: Well, Geoffrey, I think we've reached the point where we can examine the question of the social ills, and then conclude our dialogue. But let's leave this for tomorrow, shall we?

7

Socrates and Rose Discuss the Social Determinants of Health

ROSE: Are we finally going to discuss the topic that is so dear to me?

SOCRATES: Indeed, we are. As I pondered that aspect of your theory, I came up with an alternative title for your monograph.

ROSE: What title would that be?

SOCRATES: *The Little Rose Book.*[71]

ROSE: Not funny, Socrates. I do consider myself to be on the progressive left, politically-speaking, and I make a few comments in the book that reveal my inclinations, but this is still a work of science.

SOCRATES: No doubt, Geoffrey, no doubt. Nevertheless, I can't help but think that your politics have had some influence on your theory.

ROSE: I wholeheartedly disagree. I present my arguments in a most transparent way. I use epidemiological data, reason, and logic to reach my conclusions.

SOCRATES: All right, then. If you allow me to again summarize your theory, I think it goes something like this: diseases can be defined as the tail end of continuous risk factor curves. Risk factor curves shift when social conditions vary, accounting for the changing prevalence of disease. Social conditions themselves, such as income levels, occupational grade, social status, wealth distribution, and so forth, are also continuous risk factor curves that ultimately account for the majority of preventable poor health outcomes. To prevent disease in a meaningful way, we must tackle these social factors.

---

[71] A reference to *Quotations from Chairman Mao Tse-tung,* a selection of statements and excerpts of speeches by the former leader of the People's Republic of China. The book is commonly known in the West as the *Little Red Book* in reference to both its cover and the emblematic color of communism.

ROSE: A good formulation. I like it.

SOCRATES: Perhaps you were *conditioned* to liking it by your pre-existing political convictions. Louis Pasteur said that "chance favors only the prepared mind," but a mind that anticipates too much can be fooled by its observations. It seems that you were so keen on demonstrating the nefarious effects of social problems that you quickly latched on to your idea of shifting distribution curves, and you overlooked some holes in your theory.

ROSE: What holes are you talking about?

SOCRATES: Don't be upset, Geoffrey. We are both here to seek truth, aren't we? You're welcome to correct me if I'm wrong, but I'd like to draw your attention to the "prevention paradox," which you define as "**a preventive measure that brings large benefit to the population offers little to each participating individual.**"[72] According to you, this is a necessary consequence of the population approach to preventive medicine.

ROSE: Yes, that is correct.

SOCRATES: And that paradox doesn't bother you?

ROSE: You mean, logically or ethically?

SOCRATES: Actually, both, but let's focus on the logical aspect first. If the measure offers little benefit to each

---

[72] (Rose 2008, 47).

participating individual, how can the overall population benefit greatly?

ROSE: It's because small benefits add up when you consider that they apply to millions of people.

SOCRATES: But if individuals don't experience the benefits, how can these benefits even be ascertained?

ROSE: Epidemiologically, of course! We will see declines in rates of disease complications. Surely, you will agree that a man whose stroke is avoided because his blood pressure was lowered will hardly be able to experience the benefit he has received. That doesn't make the benefit any less real.

SOCRATES: I grant you that. But at the same time, not everyone in the population is headed toward a stroke. For many, the measure is a net negative if they were happier with their prior state of affairs.

ROSE: From my perspective, preventive measures will typically be minor nudges to ensure everyone is healthier. I don't think that people will mind that much.

SOCRATES: But these nudges must be imposed one way or another. They are not optional, since the whole idea is to apply the measure to the entire population.

ROSE: That's correct, but we must be very mindful of maintaining freedom of choice. I spend a number of pages at the end of my book discussing the tension between social engineering versus individual freedom.

SOCRATES: For you, this illustrates another paradox.

ROSE: Indeed. On the one hand, individual freedom of choice is paramount. In fact, I specifically state that **"the first duty of government in health promotion and environmental regulation is to protect the individual's freedom of choice."**[73] On the other hand, I also recognize that **"every attempt to change our affairs for the better must of necessity impinge on that freedom because the aim is to influence what people do."**[74]

SOCRATES: Is that a paradox or are these irreconcilable goals?

ROSE: As I said, **"we are confronted by irreconcilable opposites, yet both need to be accepted for both have authority."**[75]

SOCRATES: I'm curious about how you plan to reconcile the irreconcilable!

ROSE: Granted, this is a very complex topic, but what choice do we have? In fact, freedom of choice is at some level illusory, at least for the weak in society. As I said:

Any form of government necessarily implies a restraint on personal liberty. Unfortunately, the alternative of anarchy would be an even greater

---

[73] Ibid., 153.
[74] Ibid., 148.
[75] Ibid., 148.

threat to liberty, since the weak would no longer be protected from the strong....

The so-called free market system, which for a time now dominates political and economic thinking, implies freedom for wealth-generators at the price of severe curtailment of freedom for the rest of the population.[76]

SOCRATES: Some would argue that you are setting up a false dichotomy between economic freedom and the status of the poor. They would say that to the extent that economic freedom exists, those who stand to gain the most are the poor. That's why the poor are far richer in capitalist countries than in communist ones.[77] And, to the extent that the wealthy do impose their will on the poor in capitalist countries, that injustice usually occurs by means of governmental intervention, not because of the free market system. For example, you decry the subsidies benefitting the agricultural industry that lead to profits for large corporations and unhealthy foods for the poor,[78] but you seem to forget that those subsidies are a form of governmental intervention.

---

[76] Ibid., 152.

[77] See, for example, a recent article by economist Deirdre McCloskey in the September 2, 2016, issue of the *New York Times*, "The formula for a richer world? Equality, liberty, justice." Available at http://www.nytimes.com/2016/09/04/upshot/the-formula-for-a-richer-world-equality-liberty-justice.html accessed November 12, 2016.

[78] (Rose 2008, 152).

ROSE: That's why we need to put pressure on governments to promote healthier choices, especially because risk factors and diseases tend to cluster among the poor who will always be at a disadvantage compared to the middle and upper classes.

SOCRATES: Yet, you also admit that social reality is not strictly *determining* of individual behaviors and health outcomes. In that regard, you distance yourself from the French sociologist Emile Durkheim, whom you designate as someone holding the view that all personal outcomes are dictated by social conditions. In your opinion, Durkheim was too extreme.[79] On the other hand, you make sure that no one can accuse you of being an individualist. For example, elsewhere in the book, you jab at former Prime Minister Margaret Thatcher for holding the view that **"society does not exist, there are only individuals and families."**[80]

ROSE: Hers was a most appalling viewpoint! I can't believe that we elect governmental leaders who have such disregard for social realities!

SOCRATES: It is worth quoting you at length in the passage that immediately follows:

The problems of sick minorities are considered as though their existence were independent of the rest of society. Alcoholics, drug addicts, rioters,

---

[79] Ibid., 95. Emile Durkheim (1858-1917) was one of the founders of the field of sociology.
[80] Ibid., 129.

vandals and criminals, the obese, the handicapped, the mentally ill, the poor, the homeless, the unemployed, and the hungry, whether close at hand or in the Third world—all these are seen as problem groups, different and separate from the rest of their society.

This position conveniently exonerates the majority from any blame for the deviants, and the remedy can then be to extend charity towards them or to provide special services. This is much less demanding than to admit a need for general or socio-economic change.

...As illustrated repeatedly in earlier chapters, the deviant tail of "trouble-makers" belongs to its parent distribution.[81]

ROSE: Exactly. But where are you going with this?

SOCRATES: I find it interesting that you should lump the criminals with the sick and the handicapped. I spent most of my career as a philosopher trying to find the key to the *virtuous* life. According to you, my efforts were futile. Geography and socio-economics are all that matters!

ROSE: I don't go that far, Socrates, but I want to make people cognizant of the role these social factors play in a wide range of conditions.

SOCRATES: You will be pleased to know that your concern is being taken seriously. Some of your

---

[81] Ibid., 130.

followers have shown that one's own zip code can make a difference in life expectancy, irrespective of access to medical care![82]

ROSE: Of all people, you should be the last one to be surprised by that, Socrates.

SOCRATES: What do you mean?

ROSE: Weren't you put to death for not acknowledging the gods of Athens? Wouldn't your life have been spared had you been a citizen of Thebes or Delphi? I used your example to make the point that social circumstances matter greatly.[83]

SOCRATES: Touché, Geoffrey. On the other hand, I also *chose* to drink the hemlock, so things were not as determined as you suggest. Let me ask you point blank: Did your research shape your political philosophy?

ROSE: My political views were formed by the time I was a young adult. In that regard, I was no different from most people. But I tell you this, Socrates, nothing in my work has *challenged* my political convictions. If anything, my research has affirmed them.

SOCRATES: That's pretty much where I was going, Geoffrey. Let me take you back to the first chapter of your book, which we have not yet covered, and where

---

[82] (Chetty et al. 2016).
[83] (Rose 2008, 90).

you lay out the foundational arguments for your interest in preventive medicine.

ROSE: I didn't think there would be anything controversial there!

SOCRATES: That may be precisely why the chapter is worth examining. You start the very first paragraph of your book with a simple observation, if I may quote:

> **Few diseases are the inescapable lot of humanity, for a problem that is common in one place will usually prove to be rare somewhere else. Cervical cancer is twenty times commoner in Colombia than in Israel, 10 per cent of Indian children die before their first birthday whereas in Western countries 99 per cent of babes survive, and according to UK census figures 3.1 per cent of adults in Wales report that they are permanently sick, compared with only 1.2 per cent of residents in southeast England. There is no known biological reason why every population should not be as healthy as the best.** [84]

That last sentence seems to be a leap. Aren't there geographical or climate conditions that explain why certain populations have worse outcomes than others? Surely, you wouldn't expect mortality rates for malaria to be particularly high in Denmark!

ROSE: Superficially, you may be correct, Socrates. But not so long ago, life expectancy in Europe was similar

---

[84] Ibid., 35.

to that in Africa. Developed countries have been able to overcome their own environmental difficulties in ways developing countries have not, and much of the improvement may be due to better sociopolitical conditions. Third world countries are still far behind, and their lag may in part be a legacy of colonialism, and not because of their particular climate conditions.

SOCRATES: You end that chapter with a pithy remark which you call "The Humanitarian Argument" for preventive medicine:

It is better to be healthy than ill or dead. That is the beginning and the end of the only real argument for preventive medicine. It is sufficient.[85]

ROSE: Indeed.

SOCRATES: But, Geoffrey, if you're mortal, being dead may be the healthiest thing that could happen to you! You're not arguing for unlimited efforts to keep people alive, are you?

ROSE: I see your point. Perhaps I was over-emphatic. But what does that change? Thriving for health is still a potent argument, compared to the alternative.

SOCRATES: What do you mean by "health?" What is it to be healthy?

ROSE: Well, you're opening a can of worms, Socrates.

---

[85] Ibid., 38.

SOCRATES: You're right, I am, but you must admit that lack of clarity about health could seriously undermine the goals of preventive medicine.[86]

ROSE: I agree that the medical community has a hard time defining what health is, but that hasn't kept us from making great strides.

SOCRATES: I grant you that, although I still think that to lack a proper understanding of health is a serious shortcoming. In my days, philosophers were very careful to offer a cohesive perspective on reality. One of the major accomplishments of Hippocrates was to ground medical practice on sound philosophical principles. It would have been unthinkable to practice medicine without knowing how to define health. Nowadays, however, it seems that science and technology drive all decisions.

But let's stay on track, and let me draw attention to the second paragraph of the first chapter of your book, in which you quote Rudolf Virchow, the great German pathologist who is also considered by some to be the father of "social medicine." Here is Virchow's quote:

Epidemics appear, and often disappear without traces, when a new culture period has started; thus with leprosy, and the English sweat. The history of

---

[86] Surprising as it may be, there is no agreed upon definition of health in modern Western societies. If it is ever discussed, the topic is typically taken up by philosophers who debate the definition of health in specialized journals that are far removed from the medical mainstream.

epidemics is therefore the history of disturbances of human culture.[87]

My point is this: like Virchow, you start off your inquiry with a view that disease—and perhaps evil in general—is the result of faulty social structures. Consequently, the solution lies in improving the social structures. For Virchow, most disease was infectious or nutritional, and he could directly relate epidemics to social problems of hygiene, war, and poverty.

ROSE: Not a bad insight, if you ask me.

SOCRATES: Perhaps, but with improvements in personal hygiene, with water sanitation, and with the development of vaccines and antibiotics, infectious epidemics vanished, but low and behold, other diseases began to surface: hypertension, coronary disease, and diabetes. What's worse, those newcomers affected the rich! One could not easily invoke "disturbances of human culture." What was it, then? The wrath of God?

ROSE: Not so fast, Socrates. As the West overcame the scourge of infectious diseases, it nevertheless succumbed to the problems of affluence and "consumerism." Epidemiologists have been able to identify lifestyle risk factors that lead to these new chronic diseases: smoking, overeating, lack of exercise,

---

[87] R. Virchow, cited in (Rose 2008, 35).

etc. And these risk factors are greatly influenced by social conditions.

SOCRATES: Perhaps, but unlike the germ theory of disease, which helped identify the true cause of rabies, tuberculosis, and syphilis, risk factor theory is mired in unending controversies about bias, correlation, causation, and even the proper meaning of statistical significance.[88]

ROSE: Well, that's reality. What did you expect us to do? Sit around until we find *the ultimate* cause of heart disease?

SOCRATES: I understand your limitations. In my days, the concept of causality was much richer than it has become in the modern age, but that's another major problem we won't solve here.[89] On the other hand, you should acknowledge that the risk factor concept offers opportunities to find relationships between all kinds of variables. You, for example, have correlated social risk factors with health outcomes, which allowed you to turn Virchow's dream into reality. Isn't he the one who

---

[88] Except in the case of infectious disease, direct causal explanations are difficult to establish for most illnesses. Consequently, twentieth century medical science became almost exclusively dependent on the demonstration of statistical relationships to make causal inferences. Yet, such relationships can raise more questions than they answer.

[89] One characteristic of the modern scientific approach is the reduction of causality to efficient and material extrinsic causes. The ancient paradigm Socrates was familiar with included formal and final causes as explanations for natural phenomena.

said: "Medicine is a social science, and politics is nothing else but medicine òn a large scale?"[90]

ROSE: Yes, Virchow was the one.

SOCRATES: Then I think that you found in the risk factor concept a scientific justification for Virchow's political inclinations and yours.

ROSE: That's absurd!

SOCRATES: Then why would a person as bright as you overlook so many problems with your theory?

ROSE: And what problems are those?

SOCRATES: I think I have pointed them out already. To begin with, your view that every disease is distributed along a continuum of severity is problematic. It blurs the distinction between risk factor and disease, and this blurring can only lead to confusion. Furthermore, and as we have discussed, the exposure-risk relationship may not be sufficiently known. We keep finding out that reality is always more complex than expected. On top of that, shifting a population curve may improve certain outcomes but make others worse. Who's to decide what is best overall?

You seem to underestimate the problem of the unintended consequences of population-based interventions: a minuscule error in judgment can have massive consequences. As an illustration, some

---

[90] R. Virchow, 1848 *Die Medizinische Reform*, Quoted in (Sigerist 1941, 93).

researchers now attribute the current obesity epidemic to prior dietary policies aimed at reducing rates of heart disease.[91] Tens of thousands of children and adults may be the victims of that policy error. Another example is estrogen replacement therapy, which we have discussed. You advocated the use of estrogen by post-menopausal women to reduce osteoporosis and the risk of fractures, and others promoted it to reduce cardiovascular disease risk. But we later found that hormone therapy can increase rates of thrombosis, stroke, and some cancers. How many women were thus hurt by this public health enthusiasm for risk factor modification? Expert opinion is frequently convinced that a proposed intervention carries little risk and can reap great benefits, only to find itself dumbfounded by reality.

In terms of social and political changes, no one will dispute that poverty is the mother of all risk factors. But the remedy lies in understanding and promoting the conditions that lead to prosperity, not in minimizing the inequalities that you and many of your followers seem most preoccupied with. Social experiments to abolish inequalities have been carried out several times in the course of the twentieth century. The effects on health have been rather disastrous.

---

[91] Claims that the US dietary guidelines have played a role in the obesity epidemic are increasing. See, for example, (Marantz, Bird, and Alderman 2008).

Finally, you minimize the tension between your population strategy and the rights of individuals to live freely. You promote a utilitarian approach—"the best outcomes for the largest number"—without acknowledging the philosophical and ethical difficulties that it entails. Population-wide changes can only be achieved under the strong arm of government. I'm afraid your attempt to shift population curves is tantamount to a covert civil war.

ROSE: A civil war! That's the last thing I intended! I even said that war is the largest threat to public health![92]

SOCRATES: Then declare peace on risk factors and let doctors treat individual patients. Your enthusiasm for shifting distribution curves must be tempered. It takes faith to move mountains, but moving statistical mountains of risk factors can cause landslides, avalanches, or earthquakes! These are peoples' lives you aim to manipulate!

ROSE: Is that all you have to say?

SOCRATES: Don't be cross, Geoffrey! I am happy to give you credit for drawing attention to the shift in blood pressure distribution that occurs when populations migrate. This observation is most provocative in light of the Platt versus Pickering debate which, as I alluded to earlier, was never really settled.

---

[92] (Rose 2008, 157).

The fundamental question about the nature of hypertension remains essentially unanswered to this day. For the most part, doctors continue to behave as if Platt were right. They treat individuals whose blood pressure is above an arbitrary cut-off number as an obviously distinct population, which they are not. Public health advocates, on the other hand, view high blood pressure the way you and Pickering did, as a continuous distribution that needs to be shifted. The two approaches contradict each other. Platt and Pickering cannot both be right!

Perhaps that is why the hypertension community is now tied into a knot, unable to decide where to set the proper cut-off to diagnose hypertension, and unable to agree on the proper aim of anti-hypertensive therapy.[93] At any rate, for that insight, the medical community owes you a tip of the hat.

ROSE: Thank you Socrates, but where do I go from here?

SOCRATES: I don't decide that, Geoffrey. I'm wise enough only to ask questions. My hunch is that you will be hanging around here a little longer, and if I

---

[93] One of the most controversial topics in cardiovascular medicine in the early part of the twentieth century regards the definition of hypertension and the "target" values toward which the blood pressure should be reduced. See, for example, this article published by Harlan Krumholz, an authority on cardiovascular outcomes research, published on April 13, 2016, on the National Public Radio website: "Why It's Getting Harder To Decide When To Treat High Blood Pressure" http://www.npr.org/sections/health-shots/2016/04/13/473402142/why-its-getting-harder-to-decide-when-to-treat-high-blood-pressure/.

were you, I would take this opportunity to discuss some of your ideas about blood pressure with the man who followed in my footsteps and is considered to have been one of the greatest intellects in Western history.

ROSE: And who might that be, Socrates?

SOCRATES: Why, Aristotle the Stagirite, of course![94]

---

[94] Coming soon by the author: *Aristotle Solves the Conundrum of Hypertension.*

Epilogue

How Population Medicine is Replacing Individual Care

Geoffrey Rose's seminal contribution to public health focused attention on the relationship between disease and population-wide factors, and called for interventions at the population level to reduce socio-economic inequalities. Since Rose's *The Strategy of Preventive Medicine* was published 25 years ago, his population approach has been widely embraced and adopted beyond the realm of disease prevention. It is now promoted across the entire spectrum of medical care.

The emergence of the terms *population health* and *population medicine* demonstrates the importance that the healthcare community attaches to Rose's population approach. For example, the term "population health" appeared in the medical literature only a handful of times prior to the mid-1990s. Since then, however, the use of the term in journal articles has exploded, as illustrated in the following figure:[95]

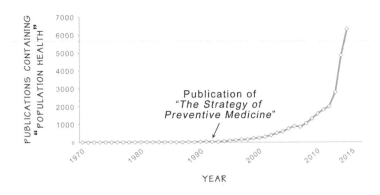

The online encyclopedia *Wikipedia* defines population health as an approach to health

> ...that aims to improve the health of an entire human population.... A priority considered important in achieving this aim is to reduce health

---

[95] The graph plots the annual number of citations in the MEDLINE database containing the search term "population health." A similarly shaped graph results from a query of the search term "population medicine."

inequities or disparities among different population groups due to, among other factors, the social determinants of health.... The Population Health concept represents a change in the focus from the individual-level, characteristic of most mainstream medicine.[96]

That definition highlights the preferred emphasis on population outcomes (as opposed to individual outcomes), and echoes Rose's concerns about the social determinants of health.

The rapid embrace of population medicine results from three developments: the economics, the science, and the ethics of healthcare.

HEALTH INSURANCE AND THE ECONOMICS OF POPULATION MEDICINE

The most important factor in the emergence of the population health movement is the fundamental change in the way medical care is paid for. This change occurred in the aftermath of World War II when governments in most Western nations began to implement schemes of collective payment for healthcare on a large scale. In many countries, this was achieved by the establishment of national health insurance programs. In the United States, specific statutes facilitated the emergence of private, employer-based health insurance, but the federal

---

[96] See https://en.wikipedia.org/wiki/Population_health accessed December 5, 2016.

government also put into place entitlement programs to pay for medical care for the elderly and the indigent.

When healthcare services are paid for by third parties—be they private or governmental—the focus of care inevitably must shift from the individual patient to the population. This occurs because the third party insurer is unable to ascertain the appropriateness of the care provided to an individual on a case by case basis. First, it is physically impossible for the insurer to muster the workforce required to monitor every single medical transaction and service. Second, there is an important subjective dimension to healthcare: an outsider looking at how Mrs. Jones is faring under the care of Dr. Smith may not rate the value of the care in the same way Mrs. Jones would. Third, individual outcomes are ruled by a potentially unlimited number of factors, known and unknown. If Mrs. Jones has an unfortunate health outcome, how can an outsider remote from the scene judge if that care was "appropriate" or not? Even an expensive investigation may not shed sufficient light on the matter.

The inability of the insurer to ascertain the appropriateness and value of individual healthcare services poses a serious problem: when the financial cost for such services is no longer shouldered by the patient, healthcare utilization quickly gets out of control, because medical care can always claim to be oriented toward the preservation or promotion of health. Many patients seek—

and many doctors recommend—greater "quantities" of care when care is inexpensively available. Indeed, the demand for and the provision of healthcare services soared after the widespread introduction of third party payment in Western countries, causing an unprecedented rise in healthcare spending.

If controlling healthcare utilization at the individual level is inherently problematic, a population-wide perspective provides the third-party payer with some hope of being able to control the situation. Rose's theory is particularly appealing to insurance and healthcare system managers, because it claims to reduce complications—and therefore expenditures—to a greater extent than can be achieved when physicians are only concerned with individual patient outcomes.

Furthermore, Rose's rationale for population medicine need not be limited to the realm of prevention. Medical treatments, too, can be evaluated by their overall benefit at the population level rather than by their effect in individual cases. To apply population methods to the realm of therapeutics, however, requires an additional theoretical construct, supplementing the one formulated by Rose for preventive medicine. This new theoretical construct is the second development that has facilitated the rise of population medicine, and it is known as *evidence-based medicine,* or EBM.

EVIDENCE-BASED MEDICINE AS THE ULTIMATE SCIENCE OF POPULATION MEDICINE

EBM emerged in the late 1980s, as Rose's theory was also maturing. The concept of evidence-based practice was ostensibly elaborated by physician-scientists to improve the quality of medical decisions.[97] Again, according to the online encyclopedia *Wikipedia*:

Evidence-based medicine (EBM) is an approach to medical practice intended to optimize decision-making by emphasizing the use of evidence from well designed and conducted research. Although all medicine based on science has some degree of empirical support, EBM goes further, classifying evidence by its epistemologic [*sic*] strength and requiring that only the strongest types (coming from meta-analyses, systematic reviews, and randomized controlled trials) can yield strong recommendations.[98]

By promoting the idea that medical decisions should primarily and preferentially be based on the results of randomized controlled trials (RTCs), meta-analyses, and

---

[97] The term "evidence-based" practice seems to have been coined by Duke University clinical scientist David Eddy. Although Eddy is known for his contributions to medical decision-making theory, it is clear that he was also a "populationist" who elevated the importance of aggregate outcomes and emphasized healthcare policy. See, for example, (Eddy 1990). The most influential architects of EBM were epidemiologists at McMaster University in Ontario, Canada, such as David Sackett and Gordon Guyatt. It is noteworthy that EBM would have emerged precisely from the country with the most centralized healthcare system.

[98] See https://en.wikipedia.org/wiki/Evidence-based_medicine accessed December 5, 2016.

systematic reviews,[99] EBM claims to make the practice of medicine more scientific and promote better outcomes for patients. These types of investigational studies are now placed at the pinnacle of methods that can increase medical knowledge.[100]

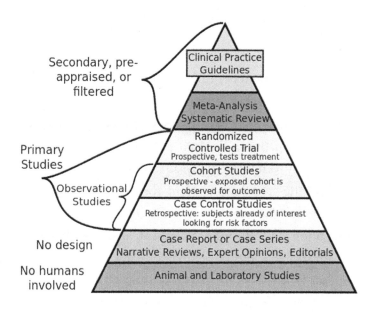

The appeal of the RCT is that it can isolate the effect of an intervention from all other potentially confounding

---

[99] Meta-analyses and systematic reviews are formal ways of analyzing two or more clinical trials to either extend or restrict the claims made on the basis of a single trial. For example, if four separate trials have been conducted to examine the effect of an antibiotic on urinary tract infections, a meta-analysis will attempt to combine the results while carefully taking into account any differences in trial design.
[100] Graphic by CFCF via *Wikimedia Commons*, CC-4.0.

variables. For example, if investigators wish to know if a given drug X "truly works" against a particular disease, they can enroll patients with the disease and divide them randomly into two groups: one that receives the drug X and a control group that receives drug Y (or a placebo). After a period of time, outcomes are collected for each group: mortality, side effects, quality of life, etc. If rates of outcomes are better in the treatment group, then they can affirm that "X is more beneficial than Y."

What proponents of EBM fail to emphasize, however, is that giving preeminence to randomized controlled trials and meta-analyses precisely moves the focus of attention from the individual patient to the population. The primary outcome of a RCT is always an *aggregate* measure: the average effect in the treatment group as opposed to the control group. It is only through aggregation and through statistical analysis applied to large groups that human outcomes can be quantified in a way that lends itself to strict scientific scrutiny. Through aggregation, one can make certain *predictions* about the effects of certain interventions and infer value about the treatment. But in the process of aggregating data, one necessarily loses sight of individuals: what is true for the group is not necessarily true for any given member of the group. And the larger the clinical trial, the less relevant its results may be to a particular patient.

Randomized control trials, then, are more properly a type of experimental epidemiology. The objects studied by EBM methods are populations, not individuals. This is manifest in the common controversies that arise regarding how to apply the results of randomized trials to individual patients. For example, to conclude that "treatment X is more beneficial than treatment Y" on the basis of a RCT necessitates making a value judgment on the *overall* effect of X. If, for example, X is better than Y at reducing *average* mortality in a population of diabetic patients, it doesn't follow that X will necessarily be the best treatment for Mr. Brown who has diabetes, even if Mr. Brown resembles the groups of patient who, *on average*, live longer while taking X. First of all, Mr. Brown may not care particularly about living longer. Secondly, he may not like the side-effects of X, especially if the benefits of X are—to him—modest. More importantly, Mr. Brown's actual outcomes are not scientifically predictable.

No individual person can be simply reduced to the handful of inclusion and exclusion criteria that form the basis of enrollment in clinical trials, and there is no objective scientific method that can overcome the reality that individual destinies invariably defy prediction. In the care of the person, clinical judgment obtained through experience and through the thoughtful application of medical knowledge derived from a variety of sources is paramount.[101] RCTs are only one source of

---

[101] Professor Kathryn Montgomery identified this work with the Aristotelian concept of *phronesis* (Montgomery 2006).

knowledge. By placing RCTs and meta-analyses at the pinnacle of the knowledge pyramid, EBM de-emphasizes the physician's personal experience and her knowledge of the patient's particular circumstances.

The appeal of EBM is that it allows predictability and management of diseases at the population level. EBM advocates take pains to instruct the medical community on how to *generalize* from the conclusions obtained by a randomized trial. But the true aim of the physician should not be to generalize as much as to "re-particularize" those findings to the care of the individual patient, as Professor Sandra Tanenbaum puts it. In a powerful rebuke to the EBM movement, Tanenbaum asserts: "EBM has remained mostly silent on the inferential leap from aggregate to individual that is required for actual clinical care."[102]

The most important argument against EBM, however, is that patients do not value physicians for their predictive abilities, particularly given that a medical prediction is never more than a statistical probability. A doctor who scientifically predicts that a patient has a 50% chance of incurring a heart attack in the next 10 years can neither be proven right nor wrong. Rather than predictions, what patients care mostly about is someone who cares about them, as Francis Peabody

---

[102] (Tanenbaum 2014).

famously remarked nearly 100 years ago.[103] Physicians should pay close attention to science, of course, but physicians must pay attention to science because they care about patients, not the other way around. EBM inverts the relationship to make medicine a scientific enterprise. Yet good medical care is not a scientific outcome.

For those committed to the central financing and planning of healthcare, however, the appeal of EBM is too strong to resist. EBM gave rise to what may be termed "guideline medicine," a proliferation of specific directives and algorithms put together by academic experts condensing up-to-date "evidence-based" knowledge. Those guidelines are allegedly designed to advise physicians on how to deal with certain medical conditions, but they are increasingly used as policy tools and mandates from insurers and healthcare system regulators to help achieve certain outcomes at the population level. The result is a relentless process of standardization and a uniformity of care that is intelligible to the central planner but is a far cry from what patients expect and deserve.

EBM has recently been identified as a type of *rule utilitarianism*: a way to provide "best outcomes for the

---

[103] Francis Weld Peabody was a Harvard professor of medicine highly regarded for his clinical research as well as his compassion toward patients. His most famous quote comes from a 1927 essay: "One of the essential qualities of the clinician is interest in humanity, for the secret of the care of the patient is in caring for the patient" (Peabody 1927).

greatest number" by blind application of a rule.[104] Utilitarianism, of course, is a moral framework that is contrary to the traditional ethical stance of the physician whose duty is first and foremost to the individual patient at hand. It is not too surprising then that the third development to come about for facilitating population medicine is the emergence of a new medical ethics that is overtly utilitarian.

THE UTILITARIAN ETHICS OF POPULATION MEDICINE

In 2012, the American College of Physicians made an explicit ethical shift when it updated its Ethics Manual.[105] In this document, a committee of ethicists wrote that while the physicians' primary duty is to their patients, they also "have obligations to society that in many ways parallel their obligations to individual patients."

One aspect of these obligations to society is:

Physicians have a responsibility to practice effective and efficient health care and to use health care resources responsibly. Parsimonious care that utilizes the most efficient means to effectively diagnose a condition and treat a patient respects the need to use resources wisely.[106]

---

[104] (Anjum and Mumford 2016).
[105] (Snyder 2012).
[106] Ibid., 86.

On the face of it, parsimonious care is certainly a laudable goal. A clinician once remarked: "I cannot be my patients' medical advocate while at the same time contribute to their bankruptcy."[107] Indeed, being mindful of the patient's financial resources is essential to good care, and the choice of treatment should ultimately be tailored to the patient's means.

A thorny problem arises, however, when medical care is paid for collectively by way of insurance and third-party payment, especially if health insurance is not uniformly available to all members of society. What is the meaning of "efficient health care" when some patients have generous employer-based insurance benefits while others have no financial subsidy? The first group, by virtue of its increased demand for and utilization of healthcare resources, will necessarily force higher prices for medical services, unless its use of medical services can be significantly curtailed by insurers or doctors. But how far should the use of healthcare be curtailed and by what criteria? Besides, doctors who treat insured patients naturally adjust the standards of care to take advantage of the expanded resources. The more expensive standards may in part be due to ethical conflicts of interests, if the doctors directly benefit from the added spending. But even if these conflicts could be curtailed, how should doctors

---

[107] Christopher Paskowski, MD, member of the Free Market Medical Association, as reported by G. Keith Smith, MD, personal communication.

determine the limits to be placed on the use of healthcare resources? There is no science of rationing that does justice to the medical needs of individual patients.

Additionally, those insured patients who use healthcare resources extensively force higher insurance premiums for other members of their insurance group who, for reason of better health or self-restraint, are more parsimonious in their demands for medical care. In the case of governmental insurance, the higher expenditures incurred by the old, sick, and frail must rightly be seen as contributing disproportionately to the national debt. By what criteria, then, should healthcare spending be adjusted to satisfy the requirement of efficiency and "cost-effectiveness" when the costs incurred by one individual are borne by others or by society in general? The response of utilitarian ethicists is that doctors should practice scientific care and their "judgments should reflect the best available evidence in the biomedical literature, including data on the cost-effectiveness of different clinical approaches."[108]

Accurate scientific care, however, is not synonymous with correct clinical care, as we learned in the previous section. Evidence-based medicine can only give insights that apply to groups, not to unique individuals within those groups. If a physician's judgment must "reflect the best available evidence in the biomedical literature," then it is no longer a *judgment* but an application of rules

---

[108] (Snyder 2012, 86).

and algorithms that favor population outcomes over individual destinies.

Furthermore, the new ethics asserts:

> Resource allocation decisions are most appropriately made at the policy level rather than entirely in the context of an individual patient-physician encounter. Ethical allocation policy is best achieved when all affected parties discuss what resources exist, to what extent they are limited, what costs attach to various benefits, and how to equitably balance all these factors.[109]

The ethicists may wish that "all affected parties discuss what resources exist" but what does the phrase *really* mean? Costs and prices for medical services are notoriously difficult to estimate within third-party payment systems, even by experts in healthcare economics.

More importantly, do the new ethicists really believe that healthcare policy can reconcile the needs of patients with the profit margin of insurance companies, the bottom line of hospital administrators, the income of practitioners, the annual reports of employers, the reelection wishes of politicians, the zeal of governmental regulators, the self-importance of academics, the confused intentions of voters, and the pocketbooks of taxpayers?

---

[109] Ibid., 90.

The admonition for "ethical allocation policy" blatantly overlooks the myriad of interest groups that partake in the healthcare system boondoggle, but the utilitarian ethicists apply pressure where they know it can be most effective and aim to weaken the physician's fiduciary duty to the patient.

POPULATION MEDICINE AS INSTRUMENT FOR AN EGALITARIAN UTOPIA

With these three developments more or less firmly in place, many academic institutions now offer programs devoted to population medicine. One such program is Harvard Medical School's Harvard Pilgrim Department of Population Medicine which describes population medicine as those "specific activities of the medical care system that, by themselves or in collaboration with partners, promote population health *beyond the goals of care of the individuals treated.*"[110] [*emphasis added*]

To say that population health should go "beyond the goals of care of the individuals treated" raises the following question: Is the meaning of health the same when applied to a population as when applied to an individual? Because a population is a collection of individuals, the health of the population should normally refer to the health of its individual members,

---

[110] See http://www.improvingpopulationhealth.org/blog/2012/06/is-population-medicine-population-health.html accessed October 12, 2016.

and there should be no reason for population medicine to promote health "beyond" the goals of individuals.

If population health advocates consider that the health of the population is distinct from the health of its members, then the goal of population medicine must fundamentally be a sociopolitical one: the achievement of an ideal society whose perfection lies outside individual aspirations. And, given the overarching concern with inequalities in the "social determinants of health," it seems that this society's ideals are founded on the principle of egalitarianism.

In that regard, the use of the word "determinant" is noteworthy. Social determinants of health refer to characteristics that are not individually *determining* in any way. For example, being black American in the United States certainly raises the probability that one will have adverse health outcomes, as social determinists may be quick to point out. But a probability is a far cry from a *determination*. Sufficient numbers of black American women and men have beaten their odds to disprove the contention that social factors are determining.[111] At the level of the individual, no cause and effect relationship can be demonstrated between social factors and health outcomes, unless one is willing to deny a person's free will and his or her ability to transcend such factors. The claim that social factors are

---

[111] For an exploration of this topic, see the works of economists Thomas Sowell and Walter E. Williams, notably (Sowell 2005) and (Williams 2011).

"determinant" also denies the value of interpersonal cooperation, mutual aid, and charity care. It invites top-down solutions to social ills, and subjugates the individual to political remedies that are ill equipped to offer care responsively or responsibly. Needless to say, the subjugation of individual prerogatives to collective action accords with the beliefs of egalitarian movements throughout history.[112]

We can now grasp that, for the population health movement, equality is not the means by which a person becomes healthy, but the means by which one recognizes a population as being "healthy." Contrary to what it may claim then, the goal of population medicine is *equality as an end in itself.* The population medicine advocate conflates inequality with injustice and wants to eliminate inequality so as to bring about a more *just* and, in his or her mind, a more healthy society. But a society is *just* only so long as it fosters *just* behaviors, and only if inequality is reduced through *just* means. Population medicine then is not only a utopian endeavor but a potentially dystopian one if it employs unjust means to pursue its ends.

What's more, egalitarianism is entirely unnatural, for it is in the nature of human beings to be unequal in

---

[112] Population medicine advocates may conceivably deny individual free will and self-determination, but if they do hold such views, they are never explicit about them. As we saw in the previous chapter, Geoffrey Rose alleges respect for individual freedom, but his own theory contradicts him.

innumerable respects. It is therefore in the nature of social relations that we should treat one another with a healthy respect for this diversity. Variability is built into biology and, in that sense, so is inequality. No theoretical construction can alter this ultimate reality. A theory of social justice cannot lead to a theory of individual health. By advocating for a forceful reduction of natural inequalities, population medicine may be particularly unhealthy for the person.

If population medicine has so far flourished, it is precisely because it has camouflaged itself as building upon our natural concepts of medicine and health, while at the same time undermining or subverting those traditional notions. But nature and reality always manage to reassert themselves, and population medicine will meet the same fate as all prior utopias. Whether its demise will come through economic pressures, scientific crises, or ethical dissidence is unclear. But fail it will, and when it does, we can hope for the return of a more natural medicine, caring for patients one individual at a time.

Bibliography

Accad, Michel, and Herbert L Fred. 2010. "On redefining hypertension." In *Texas Heart Institute Journal* 37:439-41, also available free online at http://www.ncbi.nlm.nih.gov/pmc/articles/PMC2929868/.

Anjum, Rani Lill, and Stephen D Mumford. 2016. "A philosophical argument against evidence-based policy." In *Journal of Evaluations in Clinical Practice* (Epub ahead of print) DOI: 10.1111/jep.12578.

Chetty, Raj, Michael Stepner, Sara Abraham, et al. 2016. "The association between income and life expectancy in the United States, 2001-2014." In *JAMA* 315:1750-66.

Chobanian, Aram V, George L Bakris, Henry R Black, et al. "The Seventh Report of the Joint National Committee on Prevention, Detection, Evaluation, and Treatment of High Blood Pressure." In *Hypertension* 2003, 42:1206–52.

Eddy, David. 1990. "Practice Policies—guidelines for methods." In *JAMA* 263:1839-41.

Evans Williams. 1957. "Hypertonia or uneventful high blood pressure." In *The Lancet* 273(6985):53-9.

Jungner, Gunnar, and James M Wilson. 1968. *Principles and practice of screening for disease*. Geneva: World Health Organization. Available online at http://apps.who.int/iris/bitstream/10665/37650/17/WHO_PHP_34.pdf.

Kannel, William, Thomas Dawber, Abraham Kagan, et al. 1961. "Factors of risk in the development of coronary heart disease—Six-year follow-up experience: The Framingham study." In *Annals of Internal Medicine* 55:33-50.

Marantz, Paul R, Elizabeth D Bird, and Michael H Alderman. 2008. "A call for higher standards of evidence for dietary guidelines." In *American Journal of Preventive Medicine* 34:234-40.

McManus, Chris. 1983. "Bimodality of blood pressure levels." In *Statistics in Medicine* 2:253-8.

Montgomery, Kathryn. 2006. *How Doctors Think: Clinical Judgment and the Practice of Medicine*. New York: Oxford University Press.

Peabody, Francis W. 1927. "The care of the patient." In *The Journal of the American Medical Association* 88 (12): 877–82.

Pickering, George. 1955. *High Blood Pressure*. London: J&A Churchill, Ltd.

Pickering, George. 1968. *High Blood Pressure*. 2nd edition London: J&A Churchill, Ltd.

Pickering, George. 1990. "Hypertension: definitions, natural histories, and consequences." In *Hypertension: Pathohysiology, Diagnosis, and Management*. J. Laragh, ed. New York: Raven Press.

Rose, Geoffrey. 2008. *Rose's Strategy of Preventive Medicine*. 2nd ed. New York: Oxford University Press.

Rose, Geoffrey. 1985. "Sick individuals and sick populations." In *International Journal of Epidemiology* 1985, 14: 32–38.

Rose, Geoffrey. 1981. "Strategy for prevention: Lessons from cardiovascular disease." In *British Medical Journal (Clinical Research Edition)* 1981, 282:1847-51.

Rose, Geoffrey and Simon Day. 1990. "The population mean predicts the number of deviant individuals." In *BMJ* 301:1031-4.

Rothstein, William G. 2003. *Public health and the risk factor: a history of an uneven medical revolution*. Rochester: University of Rochester Press.

Roussow, Jacques, Garner Anderson, Ross Prentice, et al. 2002. "Risks and benefits of estrogen plus progestin in healthy postmenopausal women: principal results From the Women's Health Initiative randomized controlled trial." In *JAMA* 288:321-33.

Schork, Nicholas J, Alan B Weder, and M Anthony Schork. 1990. "On the asymmetry of biological frequency distribution." In *Genetic Epidemiology* 7:427-446.

Schwartz, Lisa and Steven Woloshin. 1999. "Changing disease definitions: implications for disease prevalence. Analysis of the third National Health and Nutrition Examination Survey, 1988-1994." In *Effective Clinical Practice* 2:76-85.

Senn, Stephen J. 1990. "The mean predicts the number of deviants." In *BMJ* 301:1394.

Sigerist, Henry E. 1941. *Medicine and Human Welfare*. New Haven: Yale University Press.

Skrabanek, Peter. 1990. "The mean predicts the number of deviants." In *BMJ* 301:1393.

Snyder, Lois and the American College of Physicians Ethics, Professionalism, and Human Rights Committee. 2012. "American College of Physicians ethics manual sixth edition." In *Annals of Internal Medicine* 156:73-104.

Sowell, Thomas. 2005. *Black Rednecks and White Liberals.* New York: Encounter Books.

Swayles, JD. 1985. *Platt versus Pickering: An Episode in Recent Medical History.* London: Keynes Press [British Medical Association].

Taubes, Gary. 1998. "The (political) science of salt." In *Science* 281:898-907.

Tubiana Maurice, Ludwig E Feinendegen, Chichuan Yang C, et al. 2009. "The linear no-threshold relationship is inconsistent with radiation biologic and experimental data." In *Radiology* 251:13-22.

Tanenbaum, Sandra. 2014. "Particularism in healthcare: challenging the authority of the aggregate." In *Journal of Evaluations in Clinical Practice* 20:934-41.

Williams, Walter E. 2011. *Race and Economics: How much can be blamed on discrimination?* Stanford, CA: Hoover Institution Press.

About Green Publishing House

Green Publishing House is a Limited Liability Company dedicated to the production and global distribution of scholarly, peer-reviewed, academic books and high quality general interest trade books. Green Publishing House partners with numerous distributors to deliver valued books across multiple platforms (digital and print) at competitive costs.

The central mission of Green Publishing House is to deliver high quality digital textbooks and trade books to readers at low prices. Going digital is not only environmentally responsible and less expensive to readers, but it also offers our clients the opportunity to receive up-to-date scholarly resources on a moment's notice from millions of locations worldwide.

Made in the USA
Monee, IL
18 January 2020

20515245R00079